Advance Praise

"What a fantastic, straightforward, ~~...~~ ! As a running coach, I'll be ~~...~~ ll my runners and wannabe ~~...~~ ll the material out there on r~~...~~ d & Elite runners, while most ~~...~~ into the Slow & Steadies and Frustrated ~~...~~ Like Failures runners. The best part of this book is that it's absolutely relatable and Sarah gives you specific examples on how to overcome all those obstacles, physical and mental, that are keeping you from getting back into running or even starting. Thank you for sharing your experiences so we can pursue our dreams!"

–Lisa Pozzoni, Owner of The Running University, ChiRunning Master Instructor, RRCA Coach, NASM Certified Fitness Professional

"Running away to a calmer state of mind. Sarah captures what it means to be real. No airbrushed life here, just honesty with yourself, your body, and your mind. If you are looking for a real action plan to get moving and reinvent your running self, this book is it. Sarah's outlines the essential steps to mindfully craft an action plan to get you focused and running again."

–Amy Mulyca, Educator, Track & Field Coach

"This beautifully written, very readable book will help any returning runner start again. *From Sidelines to Start Lines* is relatable and honest. It will get you back on the road with regained confidence."

–Sabra Hawkes, USA Paralympian, Track & Field, 2008

"*From Sidelines to Start Lines* is the perfect book for anyone that wants to recommit to running but hasn't been able to do so. This book is literally your first step to finding your way back to running, or even for someone who wants to start for the first time but has reservations. The best thing about this book is that it doesn't just inspire you to run and help you understand what's been holding you back, it also gives concrete action steps in each chapter to help you get started."

–**Laura Sullivan,** High School Educator, Co-founder of The Yellow Roses Girls Club

"The book *From Sidelines to Start Lines* gives practical knowledge and it feels like Sarah is right there cheering you on. After reading this book I was empowered to look at areas of my life that need exercise and went for it."

–**Jane Trinidad-Hennes,** CEO and Certified Integrative Health Coach for Better Living with Jane.

From Sidelines to Start Lines

FROM
SIDELINES
TO
START LINES

*The Frustrated Runner's Guide
to Lacing Up for a Lifetime*

By Sarah Richardson

NEW YORK

NASHVILLE • MELBOURNE • VANCOUVER

From Sidelines to Startlines

The Frustrated Runner's Guide to Lacing Up for a Lifetime

Published in New York, New York, by Morgan James Publishing in partnership with Difference Press. Morgan James is a trademark of Morgan James, LLC.
www.MorganJamesPublishing.com

The Morgan James Speakers Group can bring authors to your live event. For more information or to book an event visit The Morgan James Speakers Group at www.TheMorganJamesSpeakersGroup.com.

ISBN 9781683505167 paperback
ISBN 9781683505174 eBook
Library of Congress Control Number: 2017905021

Cover and Interior Design by:
Chris Treccani
www.3dogcreative.net

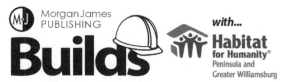

In an effort to support local communities, raise awareness and funds, Morgan James Publishing donates a percentage of all book sales for the life of each book to Habitat for Humanity Peninsula and Greater Williamsburg.

Get involved today! Visit
www.MorganJamesBuilds.com

Dedication

This book is dedicated to my husband Michael: your unconditional love and support have transformed my life beyond my wildest dreams! Thank you for being you and for allowing me to be me.

Table of Contents

Foreword

For me, running is so much more than just running. It's meditation in motion, sanity, clarity, focus, and spiritual practice.

My love affair with running started when I went out for my high school cross-country team at age fourteen. It came easily to me and was a source of fun, friendships, discipline, and freedom. Running paid for my college education, and after that, became an anchor in my life. I was a high school and college running coach for over ten years, and enjoyed having a reason not only to run daily, but also to share the sport with others.

But after my third child was born (20 years after I first became a runner) and I became a stay-at-home mom, the idea of a daily run lost its luster. For the first time in two decades, going on a daily run was not part of my "job," and I stopped running for over a year. I missed it and hated not feeling like an athlete anymore. It took a long time for me to finally resolve to become a daily runner once again. And my journey back was no walk in the park! Each attempt to get back in shape felt like an exercise in futility, self-punishment, and self-humiliation. I truly wish I had this book on my journey back to becoming a runner. It would have saved me tears, injuries, shame, and self-depreciation.

The book your hold in your hands is a tool for self-empowerment as much as it is a guide to get back into stride. I'm betting that you remember what it once felt like to be empowered by running (or another sport), and that you're ready to feel that way again. *From Sidelines to Start Lines* will invite you to look at running from a fresh perspective. You'll be empowered once again to use running, not just as a means to get in shape, but also as a way to feel alive, strong, powerful, and brave. Sarah Richardson teaches that there is far more to running than just lacing up your shoes and putting one foot in front of the other. And this is why so many runners who want to get back into the sport need to pick up this book.

Sarah and I are like-minded, sole (and soul) sisters who understand the deep personal benefits of running that go way beyond the physical health benefits. In this book, Sarah masterfully presents both the internal and external components that make up a solid running program. She highlights the all-important "Inner Game," reminding us that connecting and understanding who we are at our core, and what truly motivates us, will bring stability and consistency to a running program, which, in turn creates the type of runners that we all long to be; joyful, empowered, and consistent!

Sarah's Four Pillars of a sustainable running practice are spot on and ring true with my own "Run Yourself Happy" philosophy. Bringing Therapeutic, Experiential, Custom, and Communal qualities to your running will surely rev up motivation and keep you coming back for more. You'll *enjoy* running again, and you'll be proud of the person you are becoming.

From Sidelines to Start Lines is peppered with real life examples of how small shifts can lead to massive results. It's the perfect resource for runners who have been wondering why it used to be so easy, and now it's such a chore. It's exactly what the mid-life momma or career focused individual, ready to get off the sidelines and get back in the race, needs to get started. The simple and effective exercises will help you jump-start your practice, fall back in love with running, and recapture the consistency you've been craving.

Read this book. Drink it in. Absorb Sarah Richardson's words and wisdom. Put them into practice, and before you know it you'll be crossing the finish line feeling proud, empowered, capable, and ready for the next challenge!

Carrie Roldan

Author of *Run Yourself Happy: A five week training program to release anxiety and create space for miracles*

Introduction

Welcome, welcome, welcome! I'm so glad you are here. If you picked up this book, it means that you and I are a lot alike. You are experiencing frustration and are fed up with your running practice (or lack thereof). I can imagine that you are experiencing some longing and anxiety about getting back into running, feeling a little lonely, and really wishing you could be out there and enjoying it like you used to. You might have experienced an injury or taken time off for your career or to raise kids, and now you're ready to jump back in but don't know how to get started again. You might be feeling frustrated because it's not as easy as you thought it would be. In any case, you're ready to get off the sidelines and get back onto the start lines, and running is your chosen means!

If you truly are like me, you catch glimpses of people effortlessly running down the road and wish that you were out there, too. You watch the Olympics in amazement and wonder how they do it. When you hear folks talking about a 5K they signed up for, you wish that you could join in and be a part of their fun.

For a while I, too, was a runner who was stuck on the "outside" of the sport and desperately wanting back in. Seeing other people in action sparked a longing deep down in my inner athlete, but I didn't know how to get back into my groove. My hope is that by shedding some light on how I got back into running after a four-year hiatus, I'll inspire you to reignite your very own love affair with running, too.

It's often said that "all you need is a pair of sneakers and you can go out and run," or that "anyone can do it, it's not hard." I find these comments ridiculous and complete BS! They are totally misleading because they only apply to the population that is *already running*.

I've met so many people like me for whom running was once an incredibly important part of life. It was a source of satisfaction and provided quality "me time." It brought so much joy and pleasure! Then, for one reason or another, running fell to the wayside and was put on the back burner. Enter hiatus.

If we go back to the cliché, "All you need is a pair of sneakers," I can tell you that most struggling runners not only own a pair of running sneakers, they own many – and that still doesn't make it easier for them to get out and go for a run after a hiatus. This lie that "all you need is a pair of sneakers" causes frustration for re-entering runners and actually initiates a feeling of failure. It creates a type of self-judgment that something must be wrong with them if they're finding it so hard. And trust me, I have totally been there and experienced that firsthand – and not just once.

Through my experience and training, I've been able to fully understand why it's so stinking hard to get back into running and why frustration comes into play. I can shed light on why you're feeling disheartened, and together we can move you from that place of frustration to a place of joy.

I know the reason you're reading this is because you want that love affair with running in your life again. You want to log your miles and feel strong in your body. You crave the runners' high and the freedom it gives you. You desire your "Me Time" and the experience of regularly getting outdoors again. But most of all, you want the strength and self-confidence that you know running can bring back into your life.

I'm here to help you do just that. Let's get you off of the sidelines!

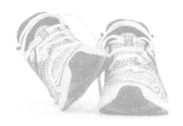

Chapter 1

Getting My A$$ off of the Sidelines

"The first wealth is health."
~Ralph Waldo Emerson

I consider myself a lifelong runner. As a child, Red Light, Green Light-1-2-3 and Capture the Flag were my favorite games because you had to run. In middle school, I started running track and cross country and continued as a three-season athlete through high school, although I was injured for part of my senior year. After high school, I continued to run 5 and 10Ks with my friends and former teammates to stay in shape and stay connected. As I got older, I became a New York State track official and loved watching high school athletes find their potential through running.

I ran my first marathon in 2005 and I fell in love! I was going through a divorce at the time and the training brought me back to life. It got me out of my head and into my body. It kept me from freaking out during my most stressful time ever! It was so awesome and kept me feeling fit and focused. Crossing that finish line was, and still is, one my proudest moments. I surrounded myself with fellow runners, and the community was a huge part of my life. Over the next few years, I crossed six more marathon finish lines and set the goal of running one full marathon in every state and on every continent.

Then, in 2013, I fell in a pothole during a night run that was part of an adventure race. I remember lying alone in the road and thinking that I had broken my ankle. I also knew that it would take less time for me to finish that leg of the race than to wait for my team to come and find me. So I got up, mangled ankle, bloody knee, and all, and kept going. I continued running on it for the remainder of the event, including one last leg the following day. I was dedicated to finishing the race with my teammates, and so I pushed through the pain. After we finished that race I had no choice but to take some time off. I was barely able to walk, much less run. As you can guess, my ankle was not broken, but it was a *mess*. It hurt so badly; I thought rest would do me good.

I consider the day after that relay race the start of my hiatus. Not only was I "resting my ankle," I also had a lot of other things going on in my life. I was getting re-married, moving to a new state, and starting a new teaching job. There was *so* much going on in my life that I focused on everything but running. I was head-over-heels in love and devoted to my teaching job, but I made excuses after excuse to avoid running in the name of "I'm healing my body." Bottom line: I didn't run. And that "rest" became a two-year dry spell. I would dabble with running, but I'd get up to two miles and my ankle would flare up, which meant I'd have to take more time off, so I continued to make excuses. I focused on my marriage, on my job, on my home.

Now here's the deal, and you can probably relate: avoiding running had a hugely negative impact on my life. Even though all of my new focuses were positive and things were going really well, I still saw the effects of not running. I gained weight. I'm talking serious weight, like 40 pounds. None of my clothes fit, and I felt raggedy and puffy. My anxiety came back full force to the point that I ended up on medication. I was totally embarrassed by how I looked, and that took a deep toll. I was depressed because I wasn't able to do things that I really loved to do. I would quickly get out of breath, so even walking or hiking seemed like a chore.

When I think back on gaining 40 pounds, having to be on anti-anxiety meds, and feeling a little depressed, it's no surprise to me that my self-esteem took a dive. The self-confidence that soared from crossing finish line after finish line disintegrated day after day for another two years. Every day that I didn't run or feel healed in my body translated into a personal failure. I wondered why my body had turned against me and had no idea how to get back. On top of that, I was not living my authentic life! My life had revolved around the fun of running. Meeting friends, running races, traveling to new places – all of that was completely gone.

After four years of living in dissatisfaction, I *had* to address this. The weight was continuing to creep up, I was distancing myself from my loving husband because I felt so shitty about my body and I was no longer satisfied with my teaching career. My greatest fear was that this was my new status quo. I was seriously freaked out when I looked in the mirror and desperately wanted to change. I had to decide if this was the trajectory I wanted to stay on or if I wanted to reclaim my life once and for all.

I chose health – and that meant I chose running.

The first thing I did was tackle my chronic injury. With the help of a chiropractor and a massage therapist, I physically healed my body. By learning and practicing proper running form, through Chi Running, I was able to move my body in a way that decreased my chance of re-injury. These external fixes helped me create a sound body again. But the real transformation came when I re-learned how to be patient with myself, and uncovered why I had put running and self-care off for so long. It was the internal work that allowed me to become consistent and fall in love with running again.

Within a year I was off of the sidelines and back onto the start lines. In fact, I crossed five half-marathon finish lines that next year and felt amazing! I wasn't back to my pre-injury condition, but I was free of dissatisfaction, off of my anxiety medicine, and covering good distance. My confidence grew mile by mile. I was consistent, and that is what mattered.

I have designed a process for re-entry that is laid out in the rest of this book. In the following chapters, we will:

- Explore common fears about re-entering running
- Explain what lies behind inconsistency and why your problem is *not* about lack of motivation
- Fully understand the foundation of a sustainable running practice, or what I call the Outer Game and the Inner Game
- Learn how to master your Inner Game
- Reveal the four key elements, or pillars, of a thriving running practice that will keep you consistent
- Lay out a vision for creating your own running plan

You are not alone. It *is* possible to reclaim your health and happiness through running!

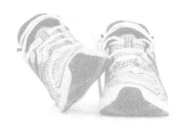

Chapter 2

Addressing Fears

"Twenty years from now you will be more disappointed by the things you didn't do than things you did."

~Mark Twain

What does fear have to do with anything? Who would be afraid to start running? Isn't it just putting one foot in front of the other? Isn't it just buying a pair of sneakers? Ohhhhh, if it were that easy! It is my experience that for athletes of all levels there is usually some type of fear involved in running. It is, after all, a sport based on failure. You can only go so far, so fast, before you fail. You either make your goal or you don't. Fear is a part of the sport, but it's what you *do* with that fear that matters.

I hear the same fears from returning runners over and over. In fact, I'll list them for you, along with stories of how those fears played out in the lives of my running clients (names have been changed to protect the innocent). These fears create symptoms that impact a runner's ability to train consistently.

You might want to grab a notebook so you can start transforming your relationship with running right now. There are prompts, questions, and activities here and throughout this book for you to ponder. I invite you to journal about and internalize them along the way to re-igniting your personal love affair with running. The following stories and scenarios can help you reflect on what might be happening right now in your own frustrating running practice. The more deeply you relate and engage, the faster you'll be off the sidelines, back in your sneakers with consistency, and crossing finish lines with confidence and joy.

Activity

Define your Big Why. Brainstorm a list of 10 (or more) reasons why you want to start running again. What will it bring to your life that you're craving? What will it allow you to do? How will it make you feel as you make headway toward your goals? Answering these questions and creating this list will come in handy when the going gets tough and you want to quit. Remember, re-entering the sport of running is not easy. You are taking on a challenging yet rewarding endeavor, so you'll want to arm yourself with the reasons you want to stick to it. Refer back to your response to this activity any time you're feeling stuck and like giving up.

Top Six Fears of Returning Runners

1. *I'm Not Good Enough/Fit Enough:*

I hear this one a lot. I know that it's tough to get out there when you're judging yourself by the cover of *Runner's World* magazine and your neighbor who trots down the road effortlessly on your way to work every day. There are *lots* of runners, but there are all *types* of runners, too, as you'll learn later in this book. Not feeling like you're good enough is a fear that will keep you sidelined. Wouldn't it be amazing to feel fit enough *now* and be free to run just because you *want* to? Wouldn't it feel delightful to ditch self-judgment and be proud your efforts? You can feel fit in your skin right now, and be good enough right now to get started!

Action Step: You can start immediately by listing five positive things about you right now. Yes, put the book down and grab your journal, an index card, or a sticky note. Write down why you are good enough. Are you already walking, biking, or hiking? Do you have a favorite workout outfit in your closet already? Have you chosen an event that you're super excited about? You are good enough already and recognizing that will enhance your running experience.

My client Julie started working with me because she wanted a different relationship with her running. She did not run during the day because she was so "embarrassed" by how she looked and how slow her pace was. She was overcome by the fear of not being good enough to be seen running. If she was forced to run during the daytime, she hid inside on her treadmill, even though she dreaded it. She confirmed that this was *not fun* for her at all, but thought that if she kept doing it until she gained confidence and lost weight, she'd be able to get outside and run at some point.

We worked on her running form, which helped her feel stronger, and addressed her self-judgment, which helped her recognize how capable and amazing she was already at that very moment. With these adjustments she got out there almost immediately. At first she opted for trails and bike paths that had less "traffic," and her joy increased significantly because she no longer felt like she had to hide. She went from being a closet runner to a proud runner by overcoming her fear! And she felt good enough to be visible.

2. *I'm Not Fast Enough/Not a Real Runner:*

This fear comes from comparing yourself to other runners or your former running self. It's easy to be impressed with runners who are fast and make it look effortless. It's also easy to reminisce about your "glory days" when you were at peak performance. It's painful to think about how different it now feels and how "slow" you are when you're trying to get back out there. I can assure you that speed does not define who you are as a runner! Pushing yourself to maintain an unrealistic pace is not only unfair to you, it also sucks any joy out of a run, and could lead to injury. Knowing that a 6-minute mile is just as far as a 16-minute mile will allow you to move forward and gain confidence.

How would it feel to know that you *are* a real runner, no matter what pace you are capable of? Claim your power! How would it feel to love and celebrate each and every time you got out there, starting today? What would it feel like to feel pride rather than shame when sharing your running stories with others? Start right this minute by writing these affirmations:

- I am a real runner
- I will make today a Glory Day by going for my run
- My Race, My Pace
- I am defined by my effort, not my speed
- Fun is more rewarding than speed

Action Step: Create as many affirmations as you can and post them around your house, in your car, and wherever else they will impact you.

When I started working with Shannon, she had never run a race before. In fact, her belief was, "I'm not a real runner and I'm not fast enough to do races." And you know my motto – I called BS on it! Speed is *not* necessary for successful running; it's a byproduct of consistent training. Being a "real" runner is a matter of getting out there and feeling good doing it. Speed is personal and something that can change with practice.

When Shannon finally understood and worked on her Inner Game, where her beliefs lay, she got past her limiting story and was able to move forward and train with confidence. It was awesome to watch her run consistently – and guess what? Her time continued to improve with each week. By the end of our training together, she ran a half-marathon (her first race ever) and LOVED it! She was really proud of her time too, and kept a pace of under 12 minutes a mile. Her transformation came from her decision to say yes to practice, patience, focus, and consistency. She believed she could do it and she did.

3. I'm Not Consistent

A "yo-yo" running plan is made up of many starts and stops over a period of time. It can be super frustrating to be stuck in this cycle. Taking inconsistent action teaches you that you're unreliable. When you stop trusting and believing in yourself, you deprive yourself of things that matter to you, like your health. Losing faith in yourself creates fear. Being consistent requires a *full* commitment. Good, bad, ugly, and slow. It doesn't matter *how* you find the time – you can be really creative.

Imagine making a decision to fully commit to your running. What would need to change in your current schedule in order to do that? Make a list of things that are getting in the way of your consistency. Think about how wonderful you would feel dedicating time to your practice. Allocating that time will allow to you to set aside your yo-yo running practice once and for all. You'll trust yourself to show up for your health day in and day out. Remember your list of whys. Start today by showing up for you and your health, even if it's only10 minutes spent walking. Commitment is about taking action.

Action Step: Grab a calendar and start tracking the days when you commit. Put a star or smiley face in the date box to show that you did it. You showed up for you. At the end of the month, evaluate if you're really committed or not. If you see gaps, assess what got in the way and recommit.

Mary came to me super frustrated and completely disheartened with her running. She would set up her training program, plug it into her calendar, get all of her gear ready, stick to it for a couple of weeks, and then let it all fall by the wayside. She was in the yo-yo phase before we met and nearing the end of her patience. She was so hard on herself and disappointed in her performance. She would rely on her stopwatch to give her feedback from her run, and when she didn't like the number, she resisted going back out and would end up falling off of her plan. Once she recognized this pattern, she adjusted how she went about her runs. She ditched her stopwatch for a leash on her dog and started to jog with him. She didn't time herself for months until she considered herself to be "sticking to her plan." This strategy worked for her and got her to finally experience so much fun on her runs that she stuck to her plan.

4. I Won't Finish

This fear is almost as common as that of coming in last. Coming in last evokes a feeling of embarrassment and shame for some. Not finishing at all evokes a feeling of failure. Beliefs like these are fed by self-doubt and negative thinking. Negative thought patterns are really just bad habits (that can be changed – and we'll talk about that). Buying into these negative thoughts puts on too much pressure, throwing struggling runners off course, and preventing them from fully investing in their training.

Wouldn't it feel incredible to know with certainty that you have properly trained for an event and don't have to even question finishing? Wouldn't it feel fabulous to cross a finish line with confidence, strength, and joy? Finding the value in the weeks and months of training prior to your event will melt any fears about finishing. Once you develop and commit to your own plan, the journey will be the important part, not any one single run. Showing up for yourself day after day will empower you, and the decision to do that will always be cherished. You will develop so much self-respect for your logged miles that the actual race will be the easy part! Even if something should happen and you don't finish, you will have months of training runs to be super proud of. And as for coming in last: who doesn't love a police escort? My goal is for you to understand that the outcome of *one* day does not define you as a runner. You are the culmination of all of your days running, and when you add them up, they equal strength, dedication, and resilience. You ROCK, regardless!

Action Step: Take a minute to define what success looks like to you. Is it covering a certain distance? Is it running a certain distance in a specific time? Is it to run consistently three days a week? Five days a week? Is it to get fresh air and have fun on your run? Once you know what your goal is, you will be able to set a realistic course of action and evaluate if your training runs are leading you in the right direction.

I worked with a duo training for a full marathon. They were both plagued by fear because they had fallen so far behind on their training program. They had done multiple marathons together before, but remembered the effort it took when they had fully trained. Their biggest fear was not finishing the race. We re-defined what finishing could look like for them. Knowing where they were in their training, we decided it made more sense for them to be gentle with their bodies, rely on proper form, and use a walk/jog technique to get them across that finish line. Once the new and realistic goals were established, their fears melted away. They had a plan in place for success, not a plan that would inevitably lead to injury and/or a DNF (Did Not Finish).

5. What If I Don't Lose Weight?

This is a biggie for a lot of people and was a huge one for me. It was not as easy for me to run at 165 pounds as it was at 125 lbs. So *intentionally* putting myself in discomfort needs to reap the reward, right? Secretly or not-so-secretly, many people are running to lose a few extra pounds. You might be one of them. Ultimately, the goal is to get in shape and stay in shape, and weight loss might be a part of that. The question is: If you don't lose a single pound from running, would you still do it? If not, then running is *not* for you! It's not that running won't lead to weight loss, but running for that reason alone will inevitably keep you in misery for a while and most likely cause you to quit. Although weight can come on seemingly fast, it most likely took longer than you think. Remember, it took me four years to "peak," so expecting to lose weight immediately is just not realistic.

Action Step: The truth is, you don't only want to lose weight; you want the *benefits* that come from losing weight. I want you to have ten reasons that are super juicy for why you *want* to lose weight. Go ahead and write these down! Maybe you want to look better in clothes, feel lighter, enjoy a day on the beach, outrun your kids playing tag, not get winded so quickly, or join that Ultimate Frisbee team. These are goals that will come much more quickly than hitting a specific number on the scale. Reaching them will be fun, easy, and inspiring, and your confidence will build regardless of weight loss. Just to let you know, my clients who find the FUN factor take action, and when they continually take action for the fun of it, weight loss becomes the natural byproduct. And by then, it doesn't even matter much – because all of the other reasons they run are so much better!

Megan came to me wanting to start running to lose weight. She used to be fit, had gained about 30 pounds, and she was motivated to lose weight – but when she ran it felt hard. She worried that it was too much work and she would not lose the weight. Once we started working together, she put far less emphasis on the weight loss and instead began focusing on her successes and how good she felt. She learned how to celebrate wins that had nothing to do with the scale. By focusing on wins, Megan was able to be more consistent and loving toward her body. She was amazed at how well she could in fact run, even though she was heavier than when she used to run. She replaced her self-doubt with self-appreciation, and the running became easier for her. She ran consistently and was able to complete her 15K race feeling strong. Her excuse and fear of not losing her weight was no longer an obstacle in her way. After Megan worked with me on her Inner Game, she replaced her worries with pride and confidence.

6. What If I Get Injured?

Many returning runners have this fear because it was an injury that sidelined them in the first place. This is completely understandable and again, I can totally relate. You remember that pothole, twisted ankle...? It was so depressing! Once injured, runners become gun-shy, wondering if it's going to happen all over again. The last thing they want to do is relive the actual physical pain of an injury, much less the frustration and negative side effects associated with taking a hiatus from running. The statistics on running injuries are staggering, making people fearful of what might happen to their bodies if they start up again. The good news is that, in most cases, learning proper form, listening to your body, and setting realistic goals can help you avoid many injuries.

Action Step: Adopt my mantra, "Heal it before you hurt it," to empower you when making decisions about your running so you feel safe and in control. Just imagine if you were able to know your body so intimately that you could ward off injury? You could problem solve on the fly and stay sound through your entire training program! It would be like your own personal super power! My goal is for you to listen and love your body so much that you wouldn't put it in jeopardy.

Rachel came to me having experienced extreme hamstring pain for months, and was sick of her yo-yo approach to training due to her nagging injury. Her fear was that if she ran, she would get injured and have to stop, and if she stopped, she would be miserable. We took a look at a lot of things, first and foremost her form. She had never received formal training on her running technique (most runners don't), and when an injury cropped up she compensated by favoring her other side, which threw her body off balance and led to further injury. It was a vicious cycle. Once we figured that out and she learned proper technique, Rachel was able to get back out there. She had her best competitive season in years and remained injury-free.

Feeling fear is normal, but letting it keep you from your running practice adds to your dissatisfaction in life. If your goal is to be on the start lines and you're struggling to do so, you will want to put these action steps into play.

If you're not sure whether what you're feeling is based on fear or fact, read on to see if you're experiencing any of the following symptoms.

Symptoms of Fear

Failure to Take Action: Avoiding running at all costs is rooted in fear, but the ego can make it look like a hundred other things. Remember my story? I was focused on a new location, a new marriage, and a new job, and failed to take action, but I told myself I had really good reasons for doing so. When you keep yourself from doing something you love, you are creating a cycle of self-deprivation. Soon you might find yourself thinking that you don't deserve to feel happy at all because you denied yourself something you loved. Fear can lead a struggling runner to experience failure in taking action.

Taking Inconsistent Action: The yo-yo running program. One day you get out there and feel great, then life gets in the way and you take a few days off. Next thing you know, a week has gone by. Or you begin running again by forcing yourself and it feels really crappy. You take a day or two off before forcing yourself out there again. I find this symptom to be really self-destructive because it gives you the illusion that you're trying, but it brings you NO joy! You are left feeling frustrated, disheartened, and like a fraud. Remember, I spent two years this way! Fears of not being good enough, fast enough, or getting injured most typically lead to this symptom.

Excuses: They come in all shapes and sizes. No time, it hurts, I had to run errands, my job is really demanding right now, I'm too heavy, I don't have anyone to go with – the list is endless. When we create excuses, it is a symptom of our fear of addressing what is *really* in the way. This book will bring a lot of clarity on why we choose this route.

Negative Self-Talk: When we say nasty things to ourselves, it perpetuates exactly what we say! When I "didn't have the time," guess what? I didn't have the time. When I was "too injured," guess what? My injury did not heal. And when I was "too heavy," guess what? I kept gaining weight and it kept getting harder! Negative self-talk is toxic and will keep you from your goals. It also keeps you operating from a fear-based mindset.

Situational Anxiety and Depression: These are also symptoms that the reluctant and fearful runner experiences. There is this longing to get out there, a chomping at the bit that is not being acted upon, and this leads to anxiety. When longings go unmet, depression sets in because we're missing out and not in true alignment with our desired goals.

Extinguish Your Symptoms of Fear

If you can identify with any of the fears and symptoms laid out in this chapter, jump for joy! Recognizing what is in our way is *always* the first step. Fears keep us from moving closer to our goals. When we allow fears to take over, we squander experiences that will bring us joy, and we totally miss out on life. From the stories above, Julie would have missed out on running outside when it was convenient for her. She would have also continued to think that she was the *only* runner like her! She fell in love with trails, and would not have experienced this if she had not addressed her fear.

Shannon would never have considered running a race if she held onto her belief that she wasn't fast enough. Fast enough for what? She was totally able to train and rock her race! She also learned how to pace herself and now feels confident training at her pace, knowing she can improve that pace over time. Speed is never an issue for her anymore. She has continued to train with local friends and participate in many 5K races.

Mary is much more confident now that she sticks to her plan. She puts far less pressure on herself when going out for a run and enjoys spending time with her four-legged friend. She no longer subscribes to her negative self-talk and for that reason she stays on track with her running plan.

And Megan? Megan has not continued to run, but her success story is incredible! She realized that running was not her sport of choice even though she kicked ass on her 15K. She had whittled her weight down and her self-confidence soared after 14 weeks of training. She immediately began salsa dancing again and has been at it for the past three years! Megan used running to deeply connect to her body, and that connection allowed her to follow her truest passion, dance. That's what I call "Running Your Life," the ability to use running as a means to finding your true self!

We can miss out on so much if we let fear get in the way. So let's remember *why* you want to get out there and run again. What will we gain once our fears are extinguished?

- Regular healthy activity
- Mood stabilization, AKA sanity!
- Increased self-esteem
- Strength and pride in your body
- "Me Time"
- Living an authentic life
- Pride in your effort
- Confidence in showing up
- Dedication and trust in your choices

Meet Yourself Where You Are

If you are ready for those outcomes, then it's time to meet yourself where you are. This is something all of my clients had in common. Each of them came to me "forcing" herself to run, and none of them were experiencing the benefits of joy, pride, and love they were desperately craving. They were finally able to look within themselves for their answers. With some information and facilitation, they all created a custom program that met their needs for the runner they were at that time. They had to be very honest with themselves in order to recognize and address the symptoms they were experiencing. Then they had to address the underlying fear that perpetuated the symptom(s). When they came at it from this perspective, with understanding and compassion, they met themselves where they were. Then they were able to move forward and commit to their running practice.

You're Not Alone

Remember that you are not alone in this. I was a fear-stricken runner who experienced all of the symptoms above and missed out on running for years because of it. I've also worked with many runners who have similar experiences and stories. They are surprised to hear they are not the only ones who feel this way. They are relieved to know it's more common than they think and that it's totally reversible. It's time to address your fears and take action despite them. For some, that means working with a coach; for others, it's finding the right running partner or group. You will feel like a winner the minute you commit to yourself and determine your course of action.

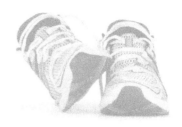

Chapter 3

It's Not an Issue of Motivation

"If you are doing your best, you will not have to worry about failure."
~Robert Hillyer

The next myth we need to dispel is that lack of motivation is why you are not out there consistently. By definition, motivation is the general desire or willingness to do something. I would venture to say that even frustrated runners have the general willingness to get out there if it could feel easier. They know the reasons they want to run again and are typically enthusiastic at the prospect of feeling good when running. When it doesn't feel good, fear rolls in and action, drive, and determination dwindle. This is what I have termed the Inner Game, because answers have to come from the inside out.

Now let's take it a step further. What if your Outer Game was spot on, meaning you had the gear, you had the training plan, you had impeccable form, and you had your schedule mapped out? What if you were totally prepared this time and it *still* didn't work? What's up with that? You may be this person. I know that I certainly was for a very long time and I was beyond fed up. It took me a long time to figure out what was happening. Are you ready to learn what's underneath that?

As a returning runner, you have the memory of running being grand – feeling the wind on your face and the freedom that came with lacing up and getting out there. Imagine connecting with those feelings rather than focusing on how hard it is. What if you could find your inner athlete's bliss and appreciate your unique joys and talents? What you have forgotten is that you were not instantly a fluent runner. It took time, dedication, and consistency to develop your practice. So rather than being an issue of motivation, what you're experiencing is an Inner Game issue. You are not allowing yourself to grow back into a fluent runner.

Four Types of Runners

I have categorized runners into four types for our purposes. The groups are distinct, and identifying your category will open up the floodgates as to why your fears and frustrations and inability to address your running issue are NOT issues of motivation! Here are the four types:

1. **Esteemed & Elite:** These are our Olympians and highly competitive athletes. Their lives revolve around the sport. They eat, drink, sleep, and breathe running! It is their career and their focus each and every day. Every decision they make is based on the benefit to their running practice. The Esteemed & Elites (Type 1) do not eat, drink, wear, or participate in things that do not support or complement their running practice. Because they desire to excel at their sport, they will not compromise or put their practice in jeopardy. Their running practice is 100% of their focus.

2. **Tried & Trues:** These are the personally competitive runners who make the sport a regular part of their life. They may have a full-time job, but they are regularly attending races or seasonally running marathons. They are continually training; it's incorporated into their lives and a part of their schedule without question. Their goal is to continue at their current level or to improve. The Tried & Trues (Type 2) thrive on consistency and the benefits that running brings to their lives. They know what serves their bodies and practice but are not as rigid as the Esteemed & Elites. Their running habits are consistent and habitual.

3. **Slow & Steadies:** These are consistent runners who are in it for the fun of it! They're out there doing races and meeting up with other runners. The competitive piece is nonexistent; they are just in it to have a good time.

(This is where I've spent most of my running career and been totally psyched about it). The Slow & Steadies (Type 3) appreciate what their bodies do for them and accept their current capabilities. They are unapologetic in their pace and LOVE their running practice, which is consistent and a source of pride.

4. **Frustrated & Feel Like a Failures:** These runners are totally frustrated and feel like failures, but want to be in one of the other groups. They desperately try to follow the advice of other runners and think it should be easy to move up the ranks, but they haven't mastered consistency. They are stuck in a cycle of yo-yo running and the more they "force" a running practice, the more they hate it and give up. The Frustrated & Feel Like a Failures (Type 4) know and want the benefits of running, but have also bought into the lie that it's as easy as lacing up and running. They feel confused and embarrassed that it is so hard for them.

Since you picked up this book, you must be a frustrated runner, a Type 4 looking for a way to get back on the start lines. What if it didn't feel hard? What if you were no longer confused? What if you could FINALLY move from a Type 4 runner to a Type 3 or even to a Type 2? Would the work be worth it? Once I figured out this next piece, I was super empowered and I felt a huge sense of relief. I hope you experience the same effect.

The Outside-In Approach to Running

Let's think back to that dreaded LIE, "All you need is a pair of sneakers...."

This is so inaccurate and just drives me nuts! It insinuates that if you have your sneakers and you're not getting out there consistently, then something is wrong with you. It makes it seem like you're not putting forth the effort and that lack of motivation is to blame.

I'm here to explain why it is *not* an issue of motivation. In fact, I can almost guarantee that you are pining and thinking about running *much* more than any other group. (Well, maybe not more than the Esteemed & Elites, but it's certainly a different type of thinking.) If you're at all like I was, you're draining your energy wondering why it's not working for you, and has never felt easy.

The Type 4 runner gets stuck. I've been there and you've been there. You might still be there. You think that signing up for a race will somehow magically catapult you across the finish line. When it doesn't work, in rolls the frustration, rooted in fear. Type 4 runners are stuck in the WANTING to get out there, and it's a mind game. Their mindset of feeling like a failure is keeping them from actually succeeding, which is not about motivation at all. This is an issue of not having the right information and support at the right time. If you're a Type 4, know that this is *not* your fault. More importantly, any Type 4 runner can be easily transformed given the correct information and support during this vulnerable time.

What I see from so many Type 4 runners is that they are going about the process of re-entry from the outside in and focusing exclusively on the Outer Game – taking advice from the Esteemed & Elite and Tried & True athletes and expecting the same results right away. They follow their training plans and eating rituals and even purchase all of the gear they are told to buy. But remember, it is easy for an Esteemed & Elite athlete to lace up and get out there, and the same is true for the Tried & True. Remember, running is a big part of their life and they are super consistent in their practice. The running habit is deeply ingrained for them, and they have full trust that they will complete their workouts. For them, it may be true that "all you need is a pair of sneakers," because everything else is already in place. There is no inner conflict on whether or not they'll get through their weekly schedule. It might be a different story for the Slow & Steadies, and it is a totally different story for the Frustrated & Feel Like a Failure group.

In general, Esteemed & Elite or Tried & True runners create the running materials and training programs available to us. Hal Higdon and Jeff Galloway are two highly decorated and popular runners who have created training programs and written books about running. They were also seriously Esteemed & Elite athletes during their day. Hal Higdon made it to the United States Olympic Trials eight times, winning four World Masters Championships. And Jeff Galloway was also a United States Olympian who has gone on to make a significant impact in the running world, and help train people for many different types of events. Both men are fantastic role models and have helped thousands of runners achieve their goals. I have used both of their training programs over the years. They worked like a charm sometimes, and they didn't work other times. Now I understand why.

When I was a Tried & True, these plans worked like a dream! Even when I was a Slow & Steady I made significant improvements using their plans. This was because we could relate in some way. I had some of the characteristics of the other two groups.

However, when I was a Frustrated & Feel Like a Failure, these plans didn't work for me at all, because they did not get ME out of my own way! Most typically, the Esteemed & Elites and Tried & Trues create programs that do not address the emotional needs of the Frustrated & Feel Like Failures. It is not a part of their everyday thought process, so it doesn't become a part of their program. The needs of a Frustrated & Feel Like a Failure are different and should include some special instruction to set them up for success – and those instructions must address the emotional side. Thus, we need to address running from the Inside Out, rather than just from the Outside In.

The following four points are must-haves for the Frustrated & Feel Like a Failure to reach consistency and find joy in running. Putting these points into action will chip away at your fears and dissolve your symptoms. If you feel frustrated and running has not been your friend for a while, it is probably because these four principles are not part of your running practice and mindset.

1. Eliminate Comparison

Competition can be a great thing and reap positive results. The following are ways that competition is positive. Competition:

- Allows you to learn from others
- Adds excitement and motivation to excel
- Helps you identify your strengths and weaknesses
- Stops complacency
- Helps you train smarter
- Allows for running together and pushing each other
- Creates accountability

While competition can be positive, it can also lead to comparison and perpetuate the feeling of frustration. If a runner enters a competitive atmosphere and begins comparing him/herself to someone else, they may not reap the benefits of the competition. There is a fine line to be walked, and knowing your inner competitor is important. It is possible that the minute you find yourself in competition with someone else you begin to compare yourself, and the self-criticism can actually decrease your self-esteem. I've seen it in clients, and I've been there myself.

By all means, compete with others if it benefits you. But compare yourself to no one but you. Knowing yourself and creating your baseline will give you your starting point. For some, you may have to walk first, or do a walk/jog combo. When you build from your starting point, your foundation is solid. You begin to build trust as you learn what you are capable of. Building upon your successes, you develop even more trust and *that* is what makes being an Esteemed & Elite or Tried & True so desirable. It's not solely the ease of their movement, it is the confidence in their movement and the mind-body connection they have, built solely on trust.

What most typical training programs are not telling you is that often *you* – your mindset and fears – get in your own way. Those training programs are not telling you that you are perfect in your struggle! I AM. You are perfect right where you are, in this moment! You are not a failure at all; in fact, you have taken a huge step to figure out what is going on so you can really dig into your running. That is an accomplishment! I invite you to stop comparing yourself to others or the runner you used to be.

2. Meet Yourself Where You Are

As I've mentioned before, meeting yourself where you are is an absolute necessity. You must know your baseline to begin developing your mind/body relationship. When your mind and your body are not on the same page, they do not trust each other. The mind sets expectations the body cannot meet, which causes failure and/or injury. And the body will not perform optimally when pushed, causing frustration. Recognizing this gap between your mind and body and getting your baseline is important.

Think about when you go to a doctor. The first things they do are poke and prod and run tests to get a baseline. Once they have a baseline, they can determine how to treat you. The baseline provides accurate information on the current health of your body. It also provides information about what is "normal" for your body. A doctor would not immediately put you on a statin to lower your cholesterol if your numbers did not reflect the necessity. A doctor would most likely start someone with high cholesterol on a specific eating and exercise plan before heading to a prescription. They would see how that impacted your body over the course of a few weeks or months and re-evaluate the numbers.

Running is no different! How can you set a course of action if you don't know your current capabilities and work from there? A coach would ask a series of questions to get a sense of your running experience and specific goals. They would not have you run a marathon if you could not run a mile. If the agreed upon goal was to run a marathon, the coach would help you increase the mileage slowly and safely, and continue to check in to see how your body is holding up. Knowing the baseline, the goals, and the impact on the body as you move toward your goal is paramount. This way you are always meeting yourself where you are.

You must have your baseline in order to know how to train. When you know what you're capable of, what is stopping you, and what your limitations are, you can get to work. If not, you'll end up frustrated and confused about why it's not working for you.

It's also a matter of knowing your knowledge gaps. Are you good at understanding how mileage increases work, but lack knowledge on how food/fuel can impact your program? What parts of a running program confuse you? What information do you resist or want to avoid? Where have you typically failed or plateaued?

For many of my clients, it's scheduling. They know how to write their training into their schedule and they want to be consistent, but their blind spot is saying no to other conflicts. Without realizing it, their inability to say no to other responsibilities, opportunities, and obligations keeps them from their success. In this way, their gap is sabotaging them.

Meeting yourself where you are initiates a respectful relationship with yourself. It will also help to keep you safe and sound. As you begin with your current capabilities, you can build upon your successes, grow your mileage, and decrease your time over an extended period. When you rush into your training and push beyond your capabilities, you set yourself up for injury. I call these the "Terrible Toos." Too far, too fast, or too intense will tax your body and it WILL rebel! When your body starts to talk to you through aches and pains, listen closely, because it is relaying an important message. It is defining your capabilities and asking you to meet it where it is.

3. Put Yourself First

The second biggest LIE that drives me crazy is that taking time for yourself is selfish. This is just *not* true! We are only as good to others as we are to ourselves. If we deplete our stores of energy, we will not be able to care for others the way that we want to or to the best of our ability. And guess what, running is a form of self-care that you need to take time for. The inner conflict of taking time for oneself is rampant in the Type 4 runner. In fact, many times this is a blind spot and they are incorrectly viewing it as a motivation issue. In reality, they are people pleasers and have a hard time putting themselves first. Does this ring a bell?

I see this a LOT! I remember working with Carol, who came in because she lost her zest for life. She wanted to have the energy she used to have when her kids were young. She was a runner before she had kids, but had kept really active with her kids as they grew up by engaging in activities other than running. Now that they had left the house, she didn't feel useful anymore. She filled up her time with taking care of other people through her job as a caregiver, and helping a few family members through chronic illnesses. What was missing: her "Me Time," a self-care regimen, and doing fun activities with her kids. She wanted to get back into running to fill this void, but was no longer in the habit of making time for herself. Now she was feeling too guilty to prioritize her needs

What Carol couldn't see was her blind spot. She forgot that even grown children look up to their parents and see them as role models. She re-learned that when she took time for herself to work out, get outdoors, and live her life doing things she loved, it was *not* a guilty pleasure. It was the exact opposite. These activities brought her back to life.

With her newfound zest, she felt confident that she was the best mom, wife, friend, and caregiver she could be. And it was from taking time for herself in the form of running, not devoting all of her time to other people's needs. She was now living from a full tank and no longer running on empty.

Action Step: Take the time to create three or four scripts you can use if or when someone questions or protests when you take time for your run. This way, you will be able to stick to your commitment by being prepared. You'll have a few fluent responses that will keep you on track with your running. For example, you could tell them that you're creating energy to best serve and love those around you! The best thing about being prepared is you may find that you never need to use those scripts because you exude confidence in your decision and commitment.

4. Commitment

Commitment is different from motivation. It is often true that people do not commit because of fear and they label it lack of motivation instead. When you are fear-ridden and feel like a failure, it's difficult to fully commit. That is different from lacking motivation and should be treated differently. In fact, you probably want nothing more than to be consistent and move up the ranks of runners, and that takes a full-on commitment. The bottom line here is that you could have all of the motivation in the world, but without commitment, you won't get anywhere.

This may not be what you want to hear, but commitment is a necessary component for you to make strides in your running program (no pun intended, but we'll keep it). Through commitment and dedication, you will progress and add distance to your runs. You will also build trust in yourself as you fully commit and practice, practice, practice. Commitment will lead you to consistency, and the consistency will lead you to your goal. If you are not fully committed, you have to figure out why. There is likely some type of fear behind it. Again, peeling back your layers and figuring out what you are fearful of is necessary before you can get started and expect progress.

Understanding why you fear commitment will help you fully commit. Could it be that you:

- feel vulnerable?
- fear missing out?
- set unrealistic expectations?
- let your past performance predict your future?

Any of these can send a re-entering runner into a tizzy and make them feel less than committed. What is absolutely necessary, though not easy, is to move through your fears and fully commit to your program. Fully commit to your goals and fully commit to YOU. When you go in half-assed or clinging to fear, it feels yucky and is not sustainable. When you don't show up fully day after day, you prove to yourself that you are inconsistent and not trustworthy.

Don't break promises to yourself. If you are truly ready to run again, you must find the respect for yourself to show up and be present. For *you* and for *you* only! No one else can do it. I can't run for you. But I can teach you how to put yourself first and commit to your goals. This is where the work is. This is the difference between wanting to be a runner and being a runner.

What I hope you learned in this chapter is that most running information comes from the Esteemed & Elite and Tried & True runners, and the gap is huge between these two groups and the Frustrated & Feel Like Failures. What is absolutely automatic and non-negotiable for an Esteemed & Elite and a Tied and True is a blind spot for a Frustrated & Feel Like a Failure.

Take this example: No one would ever question American Track and Field Sprinter Allyson Felix's training schedule or call her "selfish" for devoting all of her hours to running, cross-training, self-care, and proper fueling. No one would question it if she brought her own meals to family events before a race. I'm hypothesizing these scenarios, but you get the picture. Her habits are ingrained and are in her best interest and that of the United States. She would not feel uncomfortable or awkward giving her body what it needs down to the precise workout or calorie count. And there is a slim chance that anyone would question her behavior given her Elite status.

Compare that to Andrea, a re-entering runner who has been working full time out of her home and has to work overtime to support household expenses. She is raising two kids and doubling as their car service to get them where they need to go. She relies on quick processed foods for time's sake, when she really wants to be eating healthy. Non-runners surround Andrea, and she feels alone in her decision to start running again. She has specific challenges that an elite athlete would not have to deal with or has not dealt with for a very long time. Andrea must make lifestyle changes to fully commit to her running and that requires a different layer of support.

These two profiles are at two ends of the spectrum! And yet, that is how the running industry works. Information is passed down from the Esteemed & Elites to the Frustrated & Feel Like a Failure who does not completely identify with the intensity or have the same ingrained habits and rituals. The gap in knowledge and the fear-based mindset works against the re-entering runner and leads to yo-yo running and half-hearted commitment. I'd like to change this cycle and offer you a path to consistency that nurtures your Inner Athlete and brings her back to life.

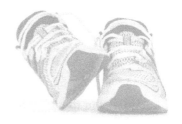

Chapter 4

The Outer Game of Running

> *"If exercise could be packed in a pill, it would be the single most widely prescribed and beneficial medication in the nation."*
>
> ~National Institute on Aging

I f you've been struggling and are looking for a training plan to re-enter, you'll want to make sure your program is comprehensive, meaning it should include both the Outer Game, which I'll cover in this chapter, and the Inner Game, which will be covered in the next two chapters. The two components combined create a stable foundation for your training and must be used in tandem. The Outer Game consists of all of the logistical and factual information needed to get your running practice underway. The Inner Game relates to all of the nagging questions that come up that create insecurity, gray lines, and self-doubt. If you deny yourself either of these components, you may not feel as jazzed about your running program as you thought you would.

The Outer Game is necessary to be well informed, but it's only half of the foundation of a sustainable running program that leads to consistency. If the program is not teaching frustrated runners how to deal with what happens emotionally, it can send a runner into overwhelm and cause them to quit.

The Outer Game is important because this information can help you jump-start your running program. This stuff is relatively easy to come by, and completely necessary for every runner from Beginner to Elite. There are countless books, training manuals, and online coaching programs that do this and do this *very* well. Runners have been around for a long time and people have been gathering data, sharing what's worked for them, researching, and creating the best running gear on the market. It all helps save you time and energy when someone else can just tell you what to do. The Outer Game is an absolute necessity for any runner, and is certainly helpful to properly prepare and get ready to go. But the Outer Game alone won't fully support your efforts.

For example, Becca was super excited to get back into running. She had purchased a book that had a training program specific for a 15K, which was her race of choice. She researched clothing and jogging bras and purchased items that felt great on her body. She thought her new sneaks were the bomb and couldn't wait to start logging her miles. She even downloaded an app so she could share her workouts! Becca meticulously worked her training into her already busy schedule and felt confident that she could do it. She felt more prepared than she'd ever felt before and thought it would be a breeze to just "show up" for her runs. When it came time for her to "show up," she was grateful for all of the pre-work she had done. With all of these Outer Game pieces in place, she could really focus on her Inner Game as she began running again.

The Outer Game of Running includes:

Training Plans: Training plans include how far you run, or for how many minutes, and on what days you should go. They may also include the intensity at which you should train. Training plans differ based on your goals. Other parts of training plans include warm ups, cool downs and tapering periods. You can easily find training plans for 5K, 10K, 15K, Half Marathon, Full Marathon and Ultra races. And you'll find that they come in Novice, Experienced, and Elite. These plans schedule your workouts so you can just "insert" them into your daily agenda. Easy peasy, right? And sure, it *is* easy to plug it into your schedule. Following it can be a whole other can of worms!

Training plans are an important part of your Outer Game because they keep you from having to re-invent the wheel. When I became a certified RRCA Distance Running Coach, we had to work on creating training plans for specific people, with specific goals and time periods for their event. It was super fun, and also time-consuming. In an effort to save you time and effort, finding an appropriate training plan is really helpful. Most plans today take into consideration the 10% rule, which keeps you safe as a returning runner. The 10% rule is a guideline stating you should never increase your mileage more that 10% each week or you risk getting injured. The last thing you want is an injury when you're trying to improve your health.

Action Step: Here are some good things to note when looking at training plans.

- Is it written for your specific type of race?
- Is it designed for your level of running?
- Does it give you enough time to reach your specific goal?
- Do you understand the language (do you know what a fartlek is?)

Running Form: An extremely important and often overlooked component of the Outer Game is proper running form technique. Think back to how you actually learned how to run. Did you have a coach? Did you read a magazine article or book? I turned to Chi Running after my chronic injuries kept me sidelined, and I was astounded at how poor my running form had become. Each injury caused me to compensate and throw off another part of my body, which is why my injuries varied during my hiatus. I was so impressed with Danny and Katherine Dreyer's approach to running form. Their goals are energy efficiency and the prevention of injury, and the result is a sound practice and longevity. Most coaches teach form in an effort to improve speed or increase distance rather than teaching proper alignment to limit the impact on your body and keep you running for a lifetime. I knew that Chi Running was a tool I needed in my toolbox and became certified to teach it to clients.

Action Step: See if there is a Chi Running clinic happening near you and sign up immediately. I assure you that you will leave with a newfound connection with your body. You will not be disappointed!

Gear: You see exercise wear all over the place! It can be overwhelming to figure out what you need, what is excess, and what is appropriate for your current goals and condition. Remember that saying, "All you need is a pair of sneakers...." And while that might be true for some, it's not universal. I remember on my drive to my teaching job a million years ago, every morning I would see this couple, probably in their 70s (people do still run in their 70s here in Vermont!), and the husband was always wearing sneakers, jeans, a golf jacket, and a baseball cap. I couldn't help noticing how adorable they were and was inspired by their low-maintenance approach to running and high level of dedication.

Purchase clothing that is appropriate for your climate and conditions, and that does not injure your body. I cannot imagine the damage running in jeans would do to my thighs! There is nothing worse than jumping in the shower after a long run and having burn marks on your chest and back from a jog bra that doesn't fit well or between your thighs from tights made from an irritating material. You'll never forget the sight of bleeding nipples on a runner who has not protected their skin appropriately. And I'm sure a blister sounds like the least of your worries after this!

Action Step: I want you to think of yourself as a running fashion model. You get to try on and flaunt the newest styles and designs. Seriously, I want you to try on everything! Learn what fabrics feel great on your skin, flaunt your figure, and are appropriate for your running conditions. Embrace your personal running style. It might be skorts with glitter or tank tops with skulls. Be your bad-ass self! Purchase high-quality items that you absolutely LOVE, they will make you smile every time you put them on!

Conditions: When we talk about conditions, it means where you're running and the implications of your ecosystem. Do you live in the desert? At high elevation? Do you live where it's super humid? Do you have to contend with hills or are you in an area that is completely flat? Does it rain all of the time? How many seasons do you experience? Just one or all four? You get the picture. The place that you run may require special training techniques or special gear to consider when you are starting out. When I first moved to Vermont, I couldn't believe how many hills there were! I used to curse my husband and ask if there was ANYTHING that was flat. I look at the "hills" I ran in New York and I chuckle thinking how naive I was! But there are considerations to make based on your conditions. Do you need a hydration pack, water bottle, or sunscreen? Do you need rain gear, headlamps, or reflective gear?

Action Step: Make a list of daily and seasonal conditions you have to contend with. Note the items you need to be fully prepared for those conditions.

Fuel: You will also come across meal plans for runners. You'll learn all about your macronutrients and micronutrients. You'll hear about carbo-loading and how much to drink. Again, this is *very* important information. Properly fueling your body will help you improve your running quickly. The saying is true: "You are what you eat." And your run will reflect what you've eaten. I remember an email I sent to my husband Mike when we were first dating. It read something like, "My run today was hard, I felt like a huge hamburger, probably because that's what I had for dinner last night."

Learning to fuel your body can be extremely beneficial. Wouldn't it be fantastic to know how specific foods can help or hurt your running and be able to choose accordingly? You absolutely can! You can become a private eye and take inventory of the foods you currently eat and determine how they make you feel. I'll never forget when I ate a whole bag of trail mix, with raisins, the day before a marathon. I had been traveling and thought it would be a great way to nourish my body. Not so much. I had to stop during my race at EIGHT port-a-potties along my 26.2 miles. I was miserable by the end of that race and learned a valuable lesson. Raisins do *not* make a good pre-race meal! Learning this prior to my event would have helped me out even more.

Action Step: As you begin running, take note of what you're eating throughout the day. Also note how you feel on a scale of 1-5, 1 being that the food made you feel light, clear, and energetic, and 5 that it drained your energy and made you feel like you needed a nap. As you see the patterns emerge, so will your super power. You will then be able to decide what to eat that makes you feel energized and stay away from foods that drain you. This information will be invaluable as you continue your running and prepare for events.

Logistics: Running logistics can look different for everyone. Are you running with a group? When do you meet? Are you training for a race? When is it? Do you have to travel there? When do you have to leave so you get there in time? This adds another level of complication to the process when all you want to do is feel good running!

Action Step: Take a good solid look at your current schedule. Where can you reasonably add in time for your runs? Note any activities that you are currently committed to that you are not in love with. How can you shift and replace them with activities you do love, including your new and improved running plan?

The reason the Outer Game is so important is because it provides you a schedule for success and makes sure that you have a level of preparation that directs you toward your goal. I encourage you to play around with your Outer Game. Take all of the action steps and see what feels the best for you. Once you have your Outer Game customized for YOU, it's time to look at your Inner Game.

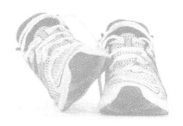

Chapter 5

Understanding the Inner Game of Running

"Our greatest battles are those within our minds."
~Frank Jameson

The Outer Game of running is all based on research and factual information. Google is great for helping you find this. What Google doesn't do is help you implement it. You can be really well prepared, but if you don't stick to a running routine, then what? This is where I've seen so many runners call it quits. They begin to beat themselves up and the negative self-talk creeps in. I have literally heard a client call herself LAZY for not sticking to the original plan at 100%. And if you knew this person, you would agree that she is the farthest thing from lazy! It broke my heart that this was the image she held for herself, and we worked to fix that lickety-split! Hence, the Inner Game.

The Inner Game of Running is how you relate the Outer Game to your life. This is the magic – or the poison – of a running program. It's poisonous when it keeps you from running, which is where you are now. I want your Inner Game to be your magic. I want it to help you find your groove and to finally get you off of the sidelines and back on those start lines!

The Inner Game of Running is *not* what you'll find in a typical training plan. They do not address the struggle of lacing up, nor take into consideration inconsistency and life getting in the way. Our way of thinking is not in their vocabulary and when asked for feedback, the answer will often be, "You don't have the right motivation." I heard this a LOT when I was stuck, but I wasn't hurting for lack of motivation – there was nothing that I wanted more than to get back out there! Still, the more I tried to *force* myself to get out there and follow a plan at 100%, the more miserable I became. I was left beating myself up emotionally. As the stress went up, so did my waistline and my anxiety medication dosage!

So here is why the Inner Game of Running is so freeing: it makes room for you to think about your running program from your perspective, not from some far-off expert's point of view. This mindset will launch you into a new relationship with your running, enabling you to train yourself inwardly and emotionally as much as outwardly and physically. THIS is the magic potion that will allow the Outer Game to become the fun and loving experience you crave.

Inner Critic

The first thing you'll have to do when you lace up again is deal with your Inner Critic. She is the little voice that tells you that you aren't good enough, fast enough, consistent enough – even that you're lazy. Your Inner Critic will also trick you into thinking that you will never be able to stick to a plan, and that you don't physically have what it takes because you might have gained weight, or don't have a "runner's body."

The Inner Critic must be addressed! We all have an Inner Critic and have a choice in how we relate to her. Her opinion is just that, an opinion, and isn't necessarily based on fact. For example, our Inner Critic might say, "You're not a runner, look at your body!" The truth is that there is no single type of "runner body." I've attended hundreds of races and have seen incredible people of all ages, body shapes, abilities, and disabilities putting forth incredible effort and finishing races with a sense of self-worth and achievement. I encourage you to look around and really see who is running. You will be surprised that is *not* just the Elite & Esteemed or the Tried & Trues. There are thousands of regular runners who are getting out there, treating their bodies with respect, and loving their practice.

A fear I breezed by earlier was about coming in last. The fear is that you're not fast enough. But guess what? Someone will always come in last. One time it was me, and there wasn't a police escort, but a Penske truck that followed my team for about 100 miles of a race. They were picking up the cones and breaking down transition stations as we were coming through them. The driver of the truck was so nice and chose to clap for us every time he saw us and I was so grateful! That was a first for me and it was actually kind of funny. Now I chuckle every time I see a Penske truck!

For me, coming in last did not matter. It mattered that my team and I covered 200 miles and had a boatload of fun doing it! Speed wasn't important. It was our sense of accomplishment and the memories that we created that weekend that mattered. Because we did not let it bother us, we geared up the following year and did *not* come in last. Had we listened to our Inner Critics, there is no way that we would have tried it again.

Ills of Comparison

The next toxic thing for re-entering runners is comparison. This means comparing yourself to others as well as comparing yourself to the runner you used to be. Let me share a couple of stories with you.

After I met my husband, we started running together. That was initially what we had in common. What I didn't know is that he had won States, won New Englands, and ran the Boston Marathon in 2:37. He literally ran twice as fast as me! Had I known, I probably would not have run with him! In fact, when I did find this out and we began to really compare notes on our running careers (remember, I was consistently a recreational runner), I became intimidated.

He would casually comment that people who walked during a workout or race were not "real" runners. He never meant this to hurt my feelings, but I allowed it to bruise my tender heart. I began to question my abilities and wonder why I couldn't be as fast as him. The more I tried to force myself to go faster, run farther, and with more intensity, the worse my workouts became. I became frustrated. This was *not* fun – no wonder I increased my rate of injury! I compared myself to a Tried & True and had no business doing that! Slow & Steady was always my sweet spot. My comparison kept me from being the runner I knew and loved.

Then, after my hiatus, it was a challenge to not compare myself to the Slow & Steady runner I used to be – running marathons for fun, picking up and going whenever I wanted without a thought. But when I had to squeeze into my spandex and still felt a little jiggly, I didn't like it. And getting winded was just unacceptable. The more I compared myself to my former runner, the less I enjoyed my runs. The less I enjoyed them, the less I ran. You get the picture. It's a slippery slope and remember, this is *not* about motivation. This is about the Ills of Comparison. It can literally sideline you.

Accepting Where You Are

This is a key component of the Inner Game and a common thread throughout this book. This is crucial for the magic to happen! So... I came in last with a Penske truck following me. I got a medal, and our team ran for 32 hours and covered 200 miles. It was a beautiful course, and I have special spaces in my heart for those teammates. So what, big deal! So... I had to squeeze into my spandex to get back out there after my hiatus. At first I was mortified and embarrassed, but I did it and kept at it. And I'm so happy I did. I truly had to accept whom I was and what my current capabilities were in order to grow.

This is an empowering process when you learn about your body. I hope you are grateful and amazed by its eagerness to work for you and heal for you. If this is a new concept for you, then you'll want to take steps to reacquaint yourself with your body.

You'll want to get an emotional baseline. Remember, this is just informational. You are not to self-judge, allow your Inner Critic to take over, or compare yourself to anyone. This is for you to understand what you're capable of. I suggest starting with a mile. Go out and see how far you can get and how long it takes you. It might be that you can only walk the mile, or that you jog it at a pace significantly different from what you used to do. That is perfectly fine! When you are finished with that, you THANK your body! And you THANK yourself for getting out there and doing it. Be grateful for what your body can do.

Once you accept where you are, you can seriously start thinking about a plan. Then when you do your research for your Outer Game, you can pick an appropriate training plan, one that meets you where you are. When you know where your body is physically, you can pick out gear that will support your needs.

At times you may have a crappy day, and a walk is all you can muster after being able to run continually for months. You also might be able to let go of the reins and run super fast if you're feeling frisky! But none of this can happen if you're not accepting who you are and valuing what your body is bringing to the table each and every day. This is so very important. You are able to meet your needs when you are in acceptance of your gifts and limitations.

Action Step: Get your baseline by using the description above and don't forget to thank yourself afterward!

Positive Self-Talk

You should be starting to see the pattern for the Inner Game. We address our Inner Critic, we stop comparing ourselves to others or our past runner, we accept who we are, we tackle our limiting beliefs, and we set boundaries. These actions will pave the way for Positive Self-Talk.

When we speak positively to ourselves, we open up possibilities. We set up the conditions for success and move toward where we ultimately want to be. I'm sure you can think of a time when you hung out with someone who was really negative. You probably left the visit feeling overwhelmed, exhausted, and totally depleted. Now think of a time when you were with that friend who is an absolute ray of sunshine and who believes everything is always hunky-dory! You leave that visit on top of the world, ready to take action, and feeling super satisfied.

What does this have to do with running? Think back to the fears of getting started again. It is easy to come into this new relationship with running with self-doubt and negative self-talk. If you talk trash to yourself, how will you feel after that run? Likely you'll feel overwhelmed, exhausted, and totally depleted. Will you want to go back out there again after that experience? Chances are slim. However, if you enter your new relationship with running with positive self-talk, you will leave that run feeling on top of the world, ready to take action again, and feeling super satisfied. I'm not sure about you, but the second option sounds a *lot* better to me!

You will need to listen to how you talk to yourself before, during, and after your runs. Are you really saying anything positive to yourself? If not, you'll want to re-frame how you are talking to yourself. You want it to be positive so you are inspired to get out there again and repeat your run! I always think of what I would say to my clients or to my best friends. If I am talking differently to myself than I would talk to my best friend, then I'm doing myself a disservice! Give yourself the BF check to make sure you're treating yourself with the same respect you would a beloved other.

Celebrations

I've been thinking about how I want to present this section and I have to chuckle, because what I really want to say is, "Celebrate like a Mother F*$#er!" I seriously do not want to offend anyone, but it's true! You have to celebrate every effort and accomplishment along the way so you can highlight, illuminate, and appreciate your progress.

I was a special educator in a public high school for 13 years, and working with those kids taught me so much. I was always in awe of and focused on what they could do, not of what they could not do. My mission was to shine the light on their talents and help them see the assets they brought to this world. I *loved* doing that and that is true for running, too. When we compare ourselves to others or our former runner self, we are unable to shine the light on our accomplishments and that stops us from making more improvements and become our healthiest selves.

Make it your job to celebrate getting out there, walking, running, staying focused, improving your time, slowing down because your body told you to – the list is endless. Every time you listen to your body and it performs the way you ask it to, CELEBRATE!

I started running Diva Half Marathons, a fabulous series of women-centered races that promote girl power, a few years ago. At first I thought it was ridiculous to wear a tutu and get a crown and boa just before crossing the finish line. But I loved the race director's mission and gave it a try. After my first race with the organization I was hooked! To celebrate my femininity at such an inclusive event (they have a generous cut-off time) was transformative! They unabashedly gave me permission to celebrate my run and I encourage you to do the same every time you lace up!

Celebrate, celebrate, celebrate!

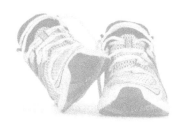

Chapter 6

Mastering Your Inner Game

"When we quiet the mind, the symphony begins."
~Anonymous

Setting Boundaries Guilt-Free!

This is one of the other top Inner Game hurdles to jump over and clear. The "not having enough time" excuse that I once used has been echoed by many of my clients over the past few years. Most people have very busy lives, have career/job responsibilities, and family/home responsibilities. This is very understandable and I completely resonate. But here is the underlying truth of that: You are only as good to others as you are to yourself.

Was I bringing the best of me to my family and job when I was 40 pounds overweight and dealing with anxiety and depression? Not really. The truth is, when we take care of ourselves first, we are in a much better position to care for others. Especially those that we love! I wanted to be the best wife/teacher/coach that I could be, and that meant taking care of *me* first. And it means the same for you, too. I give you full permission to put yourself first so you can be the best you for everyone else.

What does this have to do with boundaries? *Everything*. It is very challenging to take full care of yourself when your schedule is jam-packed with actions that serve other people's greatest good but not your own. It is time for you to start planning your own self-care – and that means saying "no" to other invitations and obligations.

It is time to start asking yourself if these things are really bringing you closer to your goals. If better health and running are two of your goals, then it's time you put them into your schedule. Your mindset needs to continue to support this obligation.

Remember, the Outer Game resources are not telling you how to say "no" to things you love with ease and grace. They are just telling you to run, and if you don't, they imply you have no willpower or lack motivation. I'm here to clarify once again that it is not a lack of willpower or motivation. It is an inner conflict you are experiencing when you have to choose between two things that you love. And you must love and choose *you* in order to nurture your relationships with other people.

One of the things I point out to my clients is the legacy they want to leave to their children or other loved ones. Do they want to leave a legacy that says they were there in body, but not always in spirit because they were over-scheduled? Do they want to leave a legacy that says they showed up to everything at the expense of their health and happiness? Do they want to leave this world exhausted and worn out because they did not put exercise, healthy habits, and self-care first? Is that the memory you want to leave?

Or would you rather lead by example and show people how you take care of yourself and can show up 100% at events with energy and zest? Wouldn't it be lovely to teach your children or those that you love how to take care of themselves so they can live happy and healthy lives? It is contagious, you know. Your actions speak volumes to those around you, and it's time you spread the word that taking care of yourself is a top priority.

I had a client who was nervous about training for a half marathon because she had a young son. She was used to being around all of the time, and was not at all in the habit of asking for help. At the end of the program, she was so grateful that she had worked with me on setting her boundaries. She was able to fit all of her runs into her schedule by asking for help and trusting that her son would be well cared for.

What she noticed most were two things. First, her husband was completely inspired by her dedication to the sport and began running more himself. In fact, on her "fun run" days, they would go to a local trail as a family to log her miles. It brings tears to my eyes to know the impact she had on her family! The second aha she had was that she did not have to be at home constantly. Her Saturday long-run days became a special bonding time for her boys. Dad and son would spend hours playing and doing what made them happy. And she was taking care of her body. She loved her "Me Time" and couldn't express how grateful she was to take that action. What a blessing to all of them. This was only made possible by her ability to set loving boundaries with her family. She declared the time she needed to invest in herself and her family responded. In reality, she brought more health and happiness into her entire nuclear family. And it did not stop there. Her extended family noticed her strength, and she received a lot of support for her efforts.

When we set loving boundaries, we all win. We get to take care of our needs and teach others how to care for their needs. If everyone on the planet did this... boy, what a wonderful world that would be!

A last word on setting boundaries. "No" is a complete sentence. If you have something to do that means a lot to you, this is very powerful. You are allowed to say no. You can still love someone and say no. You can frame it in different ways, but no means no, and by saying it when you need to, you can create the time and space you need for your running practice and self-care.

How to Tackle Limiting Beliefs

Remember the excuses we talked about in the beginning? I don't have enough time? I'm too heavy? I'm never consistent? These are examples of limiting beliefs. They keep us from achieving our goals. When we do not face these beliefs head on, we internally believe the story and nothing ever changes. It is a self-fulfilling prophecy and keeps us stuck. In fact, when we don't address them and continue to live by these statements, they do in fact become our truths. I have taught a "Rewriting

Your Truths" workshop for many years. You can find this training at: StartlinesGifts.com.

In order to address your limiting beliefs, you have to listen closely to hear what they are. They seem like truths, but really, they are stories we tell ourselves. When we want to change a limiting belief, it's a three-step process. I will lay out the process for you and then I will give an example of how the process works by using the story, "I don't have time to run" belief. This is a very common story I hear from clients *and* had told myself for years while on hiatus.

The Three-Step Process is this:

1. Recognize the limiting belief
   a. What is the story I'm telling myself?
   b. What is it that you now want in your life that this story is blocking?
   c. What is truly holding you back?
2. Deconstruct the belief
   a. Write down the actual words that are holding you back
   b. When did you first start to say this?
   c. How did it serve you at the time?
   d. Is this story or belief still serving you?
   e. What is it holding you back from achieving now?
3. Rewrite the new belief
   a. What do you want to achieve now?
   b. Create a positive statement that allows you the flexibility to achieve your desired goal.

Following this process will bring your mindset closer to your goals and foster a climate for success within you. Remember, this is not about will power or motivation. This is about the mindset with which we approach our goals. We have control over that, and when we frame things in a way that is possible, we are far more likely to follow through. Now, that's what I call magic.

Here is an example showing exactly how this process works with a specific limiting belief. The belief I held for a while during my hiatus was, "I don't have time to run." Looking back at that now, I see how absolutely ridiculous that statement is, and also recall how TRUE it felt for a brief while. This process helped me turn around my mindset, and now I have time for exercise each and every day that I choose.

<u>Recognize a limiting belief:</u> You can recognize it because something doesn't feel right. You feel frustrated or start obsessing over something. You start to sense it, but can't quite understand where the overwhelm and dissatisfaction are coming from. You can also listen to the symptoms. In my initial example of being off track with my running, I explained that I was gaining weight, experiencing low energy, and feeling anxious and unhappy. This was not who I wanted to be anymore. What I wanted was to be healthy, vibrant, energetic, and active. I wanted to be running again.

- What was the story I was telling myself: When I truly thought about my situation I had to ask what was holding me back? It was a set of words that I was listening to, "I don't have time to exercise."

- What is it that you now want in your life that this story is blocking? What I really wanted was to start running again. I knew it would unlock a bunch of things for me. I knew it would alleviate my anxiety, get rid of my depression, increase my joy, make me feel like my REAL self, and so many other things.

- What is truly holding you back? I recognized that fear was holding me back and the story that I had been saying, "I don't have time to run," was not the truth anymore. I knew that if I wanted change, I had to get to the bottom of this and understand why I made this a habit in the first place. And that led me to step number two:

Deconstruct the belief: This step will help you uncover the "story" you've been telling yourself. Until now, you have been acting upon this as if it's been the truth. It doesn't have to be your truth! For me, I acted as if I had no time to run, so I did not run. I filled my schedule with *everything but* running and it was fine… until it wasn't. The pain and frustration from NOT running became too uncomfortable to not address. I had to understand why I had chosen to do it in the first place. When we understand, we can forgive ourselves and not pine over lost time. It moves us into action and grace the minute we recognize this belief is no longer serving us.

- Write down the actual words that are holding you back: "I do not have time to run."

- When did you first start to say this? When I was injured and moved to another state, to a new job, new marriage and home. I wanted to focus on all of those things, and at the time it was appropriate.

- How did it serve you at the time? It served me by giving my body a chance to rest and heal. It also served me to focus on my new job, my new marriage (oooooo lala, so romantic!), and new home. I was borderline overwhelmed with all of that transition. I had all of that going on, and the last thing I wanted to do was pack an extra bag, stop at a new gym, and meet even more new people. I really wanted to master what I had going on in that moment and not spread myself too thin. And my body really did need to heal.

- Is this story or belief still serving you? No, not at all! Four years later, that story had become a bad habit and was no longer serving me. I was settled with my new business and my marriage was superb, but my weight gain had actually caused a decrease in the ooooooo lala romance, if you get my drift. I really wanted my old body back, I wanted to get off my anxiety medicine and knew that running was the action I needed to take.

- What is it holding you back from achieving now? I realized that my *words* and mindset were holding me back. I had to adjust my thinking. I *did* have time, but when I told myself I didn't, and it was now solidly ingrained, I acted upon that as it were the truth.

<u>Rewrite the new belief</u>:

- What do you want to achieve now? I wanted time to run!
- Create a positive statement that allows you flexibility to achieve your desired goal. The statement, new truth, and new beliefs I set were positive *and* allowed for flexibility and worked like a charm. I changed my old belief to, "I have plenty of time during the day to do whatever is best for me and everyone involved." Let me explain this statement. You'll notice that it is NOT, "I have time to run every day." I could have easily said that but I knew it would set me up for an all-or-nothing attitude. If I missed a day, I would beat myself up. This statement left me open to choose to have the time to run and, more often, I did. And I did not feel guilty if I had some other responsibility come up and couldn't go. This statement was truly freeing and helped me move toward my goal with a positive outlook.

If you have any questions about this process or need help coming up with a re-frame for your wording, email me immediately! I want to help you get out of your own way with your thinking. This is super important and we can get you on a path to success lickety-split!

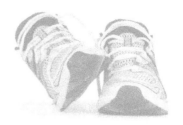

Chapter 7

Embrace the Four Pillars of a Sustainable Running Practice

"The real voyage of discovery consists not in seeking new landscapes, but in seeing with new eyes."
~Marcel Proust

T he four pillars of a sustainable running practice are:
- Therapeutic
- Experiential
- Custom
- Communal

These four components work in concert to create a solid structure for a practice that lights you up. They fulfill your why, and keep you coming back for more day after day. I call them the pillars of the practice because when these four components are solidly in place and a part of your running mindset, your practice becomes *fun* and super beneficial for you.

The pillars work as the support system of any running program and provide a guideline for creating your practice. All components must be present for you to fully connect to your running and receive the full benefits. Your four pillars transform daily runs into a journey of a lifetime. It is how your inner joy is expressed through the outward act of running. I live by these pillars and bring them whole-heartedly into my coaching programs. When running is just based on burning calories, or to lose weight, or, worse yet, as just a "thing on the to-do list," you'll never find your mojo, and consistency will continue to be an issue.

Running as Therapy

> *"Running should be a relief from stress, a way to cope with it, not another added stress."*
> ~ Bob Glover

> *"I have two doctors: my left leg and my right."*
> ~ George M. Trevelyan

Therapy by definition is: o*f or relating to the healing of disease*. This is completely true for running. When you add a form of exercise to your life, you receive so many physical *and* emotional benefits. For example, you'll reduce your blood pressure, decrease your chances for heart disease, increase your lifespan, and improve your brain performance. If that's not enough for you, running can help you sleep better, improve your mood, and improve your self-esteem. I'm sure this is why being on the sidelines has been so frustrating and stress-producing for you!

Here is an awesome conversation starter I heard from someone a few weeks ago. He knew I was a running coach and he said, "I heard that people who run are usually running away from things, but they're also running toward things." It was the start of a wonderful conversation. This *is* what makes running so therapeutic! Everyone has issues, problems that crop up and at times we don't want to deal with them. Running is a great way to burn off the anxiety created by any situation. Frequently, by the time you get back from your run (which is a long series of deep breathing exercises, if we're being honest), you'll feel like there is no problem or issue any more. Most likely you've solved your problem, came up with a creative solution, or just feel so relaxed and accomplished that whatever was bugging you just doesn't matter any more! Running is truly a win-win situation for this reason. It allows you to run away from the problem and to a calmer state of mind. Running marathons got me through a two-year long divorce! If that isn't therapeutic, I don't know what is!

I don't have to sell you on running being therapeutic, I'm sure it is a major reason why you want to reclaim your practice. Which of the following reasons do you find running therapeutic?

"Me Time." We talked about this earlier, how getting some alone time can be a precious commodity in this day and age. You get to think and sort out your own thoughts. You get to celebrate your body movement (don't you dare forget to celebrate!). You also get to leave behind the pressures of life and do your own thing during your run. You can be fully present for yourself and leave your worries elsewhere.

Action Step: How about starting right now by picking a regular "Me Time" and adding it to your calendar?

Sanity. Most people are super busy and overly committed. Running clears the mind and allows sanity and focus to roll in. Remember my story: I was on anti-anxiety meds for four years, but that's all ancient history now that running has re-entered my life. Now, if my eye starts to twitch, I know I'm feeling stressed and I can go for a jog and calm down. Enter sanity! Are you ready to leave behind the hustle and the rat race and allow some clarity and calm to come in?

Action Step: Switch out saying yes to something you feel "obligated" to do and say yes to yourself and go for a jog. Sanity will seep in!

Mind/Body Connection: Another challenge that re-entering runners face is that they lack meaningful connection between their mind and their body, often to the point of distrust. The saying "no pain no gain" is a stunning example of how to create distrust. Would you stick around if someone hit you? Would you encourage abusive relationships? I certainly doubt it! Pushing through an injury is very similar, except it is you who is abusing your body. When you run, and deeply listen to your body and feel for the messages it sends, you nourish your mind/body relationship. It is therapeutic because if you are connected to your body, you are able to listen to any pangs and autocorrect.

Action Step: Today, be open to the messages your body is sending you. Are you feeling tired? Achy? Are you excited or happy? Make note of these messages and what triggered them. Sort and list them into two groups, positive and negative, so you can refer back to your specific actions that initiated a positive response versus a negative response.

Reboot: Aka, de-stress. A run can reboot your thought processes and take you out of the mind block that comes with overwhelm. My husband is a daily runner; he runs during lunch at work. He will always tell his team he is going to therapy and he'll be back in an hour. He swears that his continued productivity and focus are benefits of his midday run. It allows him to breathe in fresh air, clear his blood, and finish his workday as strong as he started.

Action Step: Are there times in your day or in your life when you need a reboot? Is your job stressful? Is your home life stressful? Do particular times of the year bring on excess stress? Take an inventory of stressful times and plan to use your running as a reboot.

Social Hour: There are "Me Time" runs and there are social hour runs. Some people mix it up depending on the day. Runners are awesome and some of the most supportive people on the planet. It's fun to get out and chat with your friends as you cover the miles. My running mates and I joke about how we solve the problems of the world by the end of our runs!

Action Step: Imagine that instead of reaching for that ice cold beer at the end of the day with your friend or that Sunday brunch buffet with your family, you met up with another runner or group of runners instead to chit chat away? List the family members, friends, or local running groups that could replace over-indulgent social hours with a fun and healthy social hour.

Flush Out Toxins: Cardiovascular exercise is notorious for increasing your blood flow, which floods oxygen to your system. This helps your organs work optimally and escorts toxins out of your body! Whooo hoooo!

Action Step: Burn baby burn! Celebrate that every time you are out there, you are making strides toward your clean and healthy body! Remember that calendar you set up with your stars or smiley faces? You can also record your time, distance, and calorie burn if you want.

The therapeutic qualities of running are many, but they are sometimes not externally obvious. It's not easy to "see" blood pressure go down; it takes a while to lose unwanted weight, and there might still be things that trigger anxiety and depression. The mind/body connection is the important piece to keep in mind. As you integrate running into your life, focus on remembering all of the physical benefits you are initiating. You are protecting yourself from disease; you are limiting the impact that emotional stress can have on you. Don't forget to check in with your top 10 reasons for running that you came up with at the beginning of the book. Over time you WILL begin to notice, if you are connecting your mind and body, the positive physical and emotional impact on your body. And when these results become apparent, you will enjoy your practice all the more!

Let's reconnect with Mary. She came to me hating her running program and was not seeing the "results" she was looking for. She was running three or four days a week, meeting her mileage goal, and running for time. She never left her house without her Fitbit and stop watch and was rigid with her training program. If she was sick and missed a day, her inner critic would immediately start berating her for being such a slacker. Her motto was to push through and force her workouts come hell or high water! Needless to say, Mary was majorly disappointed with her running.

I asked her if she enjoyed it. She said no. So why do you do it? She said to lose weight. I asked her what benefits she got from it, and she didn't have an answer. Her attachment was not to any of the health benefits or therapeutic qualities. She was missing out on such a huge component of running! When she switched her mindset, ditched her watch, headed out into nature, and used her runs as a way to reboot after a long day at work, she began to enjoy it more. I loved seeing her smile as she began to talk about her runs! Then she began to bring her dog and got some needed bonding time with him. Her runs became purposeful and shifted from a check on her to-do list to a quality "Me Time" practice where she could be at peace with her body. *That* was a huge shift! Over time she became more consistent and the weight loss was a byproduct of a consistent practice. That is therapy!

Running Is Experiential

> *"I frequently tramped eight or ten miles through the deepest snow to keep an appointment with a beech tree, or a yellow birch, or an old acquaintance among the pines."*
> ~Henry David Thoreau

Making It Fun

Making your run FUN is the whole point. Mary's stop watch was a great tool for a while until it became her only focus. She had to take her runs to different places and focus on her experience versus her performance. You can only take so much self-judgment before you just give up!

I have always prided myself on seeing the glory of this beautiful planet we are blessed to inhabit. I love the colors in Fall (as I'm writing this book, the leaves are on fire outside), the quiet of winter when there is a blanket of snow, the stickiness of the mud and the joy of longer days in the spring, and the smell of cut grass and the feel of the sunshine on my skin during the summer. Getting out there to enjoy these gems year round are gifts specially delivered to us from Mother Nature! What a concept: to make the focus pure enjoyment of the world surrounding us!

Embrace Your Place

As you learn to embrace your place, you can appreciate even the man-made additions to our world. Have you ever gone to a city, listen to the sounds, smelled the smells? You can "embrace your place," get a sense of the community, and see it from a whole different perspective. Years ago, running through Athens, Greece gave me a feeling of pride, especially going past the Olympic Stadium. To see those iconic overlapping circles and think about the elite athletes who ran that track was amazing. I also watched locals walking on their way to and from work or on errands. I noticed what they wore, what they carried, and if they smiled and returned my hello. I read storefront signs and could see the Acropolis rise up behind some of the buildings. What was it like to have lived here "back in the day?" My mind wandered and I covered ground admiring the democratic traditions that were birthed right here on this soil. It was amazing. Stop watch – no way! Beating myself up – not a chance! Forty-minute run completed in what seemed like two minutes – hell, yeah! Memories created for a lifetime – yes and amen!

Action Step: What beauty and fresh perspective can you gain from your current surroundings? Where can you choose to run that will give you an experiential outcome? Take pictures of the beauty you see, the things that crack you up or surprise you. Take inventory of your surroundings and create this habit that can apply to all parts of your life!

Ditch Technology

Technology has its time and place, but it can also become a distraction. If relied on too heavily, it can sever your mind-body relationship. When you ditch technology, and I'm talking watches, timers, trackers, etc., your blinders come off. Your run becomes limitless and free of judgment. It's just you, your body, and your surroundings. You get to create the experience you *want!* You engage with your environment rather than with your technical devices. Let go of time, let go of pace, calorie burn, let go of expectations, and enjoy the scenery!

Give yourself permission to stop and take a picture of a beautiful vista, pretty plant, or ray of sunshine cutting through the woods. Allow yourself to stop and window shop if you see something striking that catches your eye. It's all OK if you are enjoying each and every step of the way. Guess what, this can even be true on a treadmill! Try it: Forego the timers, lap counters, and intensity charts. Cover up the gauges with a magazine and let your mind connect to your body in its entirety. Feel how your feet are falling, count your breath, feel your diaphragm going in and out. If you're in a gym, you can TOTALLY people watch! It doesn't have to be boring on a treadmill! Allow your mind to wander and solve your problems! Turn your "dreadmill" experience into a therapeutic and experiential one!

Action Step: Forego your technology for tracking purposes one day a week and record what you notice. I do encourage you to bring your cell phone for safety purposes (and picture-taking), but resist the temptation to use it to track your stats on every run.

Use Your Senses

We have five senses. When was the last time you actually *used* them with intention? Do you take them for granted? Sight, sound, touch, taste, and smell. These are gifts we should be enjoying and that contribute to the experiential nature of our lives. When you use your senses, you'll be brought back to places over and over during your lifetime because your senses will trigger nostalgic memories.

Take some time to be mindful of what you're seeing. Just look around and take in the sights. Your ears also play a part in your running. Sometimes it can be really loud when you're out there. What's making the noise? Airplanes? Traffic? Barking dogs? When you focus on what you hear, you are more alert. If it's quiet, can you hear your breath? Your footfalls? Bugs or birds?

Touch and taste may seem like difficult senses to connect with when you're running but I can assure you that it's possible! Can you feel the humidity in the air or is it crisp? Can you feel the sun on your skin or the wind in your hair? Can you feel the water splashing up from puddles? There is so much to touch and feel! And as for taste, can you taste the salt in the air near an ocean? Can you taste the arid heat in a desert? Can you taste the sweat from your lip or the polluted air in a city? Bring awareness to your taste. As you move to smell, you can think about running in NYC during the winter and smelling the roasting chestnuts on each corner, or the smell of the Green Mountain Coffee Roasters plant as you jog by their campus in Vermont. Sipping your morning coffee will bring you back to that jog.

I had the great pleasure of training with Danny Dreyer, the co-founder of Chi Running, and he brought us on one of my favorite runs of all time. We went for a 30-minute run and set a stopwatch to beep every six minutes. For each of the five intervals, we would switch our focus to a different sense. I was amazed at how incredibly easy and fast that run went! We seemed to just float through the trails. I can specifically recall the experience I had with each sense. And it was just by making the run experiential that brought ease and grace to that workout.

Action Step: Use all five of your senses today. Note what came up for you and if you experienced any nostalgia.

The Experience of a Race

Races aren't for everyone, but they are certainly an experience! Races come in all different distances, from one-milers to Ultras (anything over 26.2 miles). They can be done alone or as teams. They can be highly competitive or total fun runs. You can make a race your own experience. I have met some of the most inspiring people at races. I've also felt the most fear at races. The mixed bag of emotions is bottomless!

I remember getting on the starting line with Shannon, who was afraid she wasn't good enough or fast enough when we started working together. It was her first race ever, and it was a half marathon. We both choked up as they played the national anthem. She was still slightly fearful of the time cut-off and her ability to finish, but her biggest emotion was excitement beyond belief. She was eased by the lightheartedness of the race, donning a tutu, tiara, and boa. She found her feminine confidence as she was enveloped into a sea of pink! Her experience was glorious! Her adrenaline carried her the 13.1 miles, and her preparation did not fail her. She flowed over the hilly course and beat her average pace by ten seconds per mile. Her first race washed away all fear of competition! She loved the camaraderie, the shared experience of all, and the accomplishment of the women who surrounded her. It wasn't a week later that she was on the start line of a 5K and sharing how much fun THAT one was for her too!

Action Step: Is it time for you to cross a finish line again? That IS why you're reading, right? Not in a competitive way, but in a way that will make you feel like you're "in the game again." Look at your schedule and look at upcoming races that you are interested in. Please note finish times, are they open to walkers? Set yourself up for success and take action! As you register for this race, you may be triggered with some fears. Go back and use this book to problem-solve your fear or reach out to me for more structured support!

Beyond Running

If you want to challenge yourself a little more and treat your Inner Athlete to something a little different, there are all types of adventure races now that are accessible to multiple levels of athletes. There are races like Spartan Races, which are typically associated with hard-core runners who cross train a lot. But the Dirty Girl Mud Races are super fun and are an adventure in themselves. Yes, you do need some athletic ability, but these are far less competitive than the Spartan Races and geared toward being fun and accessible for athletes of all levels. If plain old running turns boring for you, try an adventure race to spruce it up. It's a great way to keep your running experiential.

Run Your Life

It is amazing how creating space in our schedule for running and carving out time for self-care begins to open doors in other parts of life, too. Have you noticed that the world can become your oyster? You create fertile ground when you take control of your actions and invest in your decision to start to running. The bigger benefit of focusing your time and investing your energy is that the same skill can be used for acquiring anything in your life! Commitment here will lead to commitment and achievements in other areas of your life.

For example, when purchasing a house, you'll use the same skills. You'll have to carve out time in your schedule for appointments to see houses, meet with banks, and go over paperwork. You may even choose to work additional hours to save money for your down payment. You will save diligently to build your nest egg, knowing that every penny counts. You will be patient and make consistent decisions to cut spending in order to make your down payment. You'll be setting lots of loving boundaries as this venture takes time away from other things and people, and you'll have to use self-discipline daily to make decisions that bring you closer to owning a house.

When you set an intention and you stick to your plan, you will reach your goal. Wha-La. You just used the same method we talked about for integrating running into your life. Hence, you can now Run Your Life, because you have the skills necessary to see your intentions, clear room in your schedule to work toward it, take action and achieve it! Superb!

Action Step: Take a few minutes and journal about other areas of your life that need attention and focus. What have you been tolerating in your life that would feel freeing to address? Is there some organizing that you've been meaning to do or paperwork that needs to be done? What things have been on the back burner and would make you feel lighter for taking care of them? Jot down a few things and keep them in mind. Once you have solidified your running, see if you are able to check anything else off of this list.

Run the World

I caught the "Travel Bug" when I was young. And being a runner, I took it everywhere I traveled. Before my four-year hiatus, I would pick marathons and races across the globe and make the training more meaningful because at the end was the reward of a fabulous vacation. My first marathon was in Honolulu, and it was a trip I took with my best friend Leanne. I remember how exciting it was, and the fulfillment of crossing that finish line. That trip that I took with Leanne changed not only my life, but her life, too. She had not been a runner, but my best cheerleader as I embarked on that journey.

The day before the race, at the expo, she signed up for the 10K walk. It was my first marathon and her first event, and we were so excited and nervous! Race day was like a dream. We both did something we had never done before! Talk about celebration! We both were in the clouds, figuratively, for being so proud of our accomplishments – and then literally, because the next day we hiked Diamond Head. What an experience!

Again, my goal is for all of this to be transferrable to your everyday life. When you go on a family vacation, why not check out the local scene by foot?

I remember one morning in Spain with my friends Laura and Mo. I got up early and hit the streets for some "Me Time" and exploration. I found a park in San Sebastian overlooking the Bay of Biscay, and it was spectacular. Before heading back, I stopped by the train station and picked up tickets for us to go to Pamplona for the running of the bulls. I'll never forget the excitement as I tucked those tickets in my pouch and headed back to our room. We did not run with the bulls (that's a little too risky), but we spent the night in town witnessing the ancient tradition and experiencing Spanish culture. Running helped me deepen my experience in Spain.

So imagine YOU getting out there and having the time of YOUR life training for an event, and loving the experience of each run. Imagine reaping all of the therapeutic qualities that running provides your mind, body, and soul. Imagine the pride and confidence it would give you! Where would you love to travel? Would that be enough of a reward for you to commit?

Action Step: Dream of crossing that finish line! Dream of your success! Dream of your CELEBRATION! What would it look like? Describe it in your journal. If there were a race anywhere in the world that you want to do, email it to me at Sarah@RiseAndShine.Run. I totally want to know! Maybe we can turn it into a racecation!

Running Is Custom

"Running gives you freedom. When you run, you can go at your own speed. You can go where you want to go and think your own thought. Nobody has any claim on you."

~ Nina Kuscsik

Your dream WILL come true, but you must adhere to the third pillar of a successful running practice and make sure it's customized for *you*. Remember in Chapter 4 where we spoke about accepting where you are? This is where that gets put into practice. It's awesome if you find a training program for a Half Marathon, but when you customize it to meet all of your needs, that's a win-win.

There are so many factors that impact the right plan for YOU: your past experience, your upcoming goals, your current level of physical fitness, your support system, your location and climate, your current responsibilities and obligations, your specific frustrations, past injuries… the list goes on. No wonder you were frustrated and overwhelmed! Everyone is so very different. It would be naïve to think that that one plan fits all. And it is probably what led you to this book. The Outer Game that you tried did not fully meet your needs. It wasn't enough support for your Inner Game. Here are some things to keep in mind as you customize your running plan. There will be action steps for each item.

You Are YOU

You are unique. Your tastes and talents are your own! Your capabilities and your preferences are unique to you. To be unapologetically yourself may take some practice, but once you do it, you'll *never* go back! As a coach, people often look to me as an authority of some sort. They want me to tell them what to do, because that seems easy and they trust that what I say will work for them. As a coach I truly believe that you know yourself best and as I get to know you, I can develop a plan *with* you that completely suits your needs. When I co-create plans with my clients, sustainability and success increase.

Think about the beloved diet book. There are thousands of them out there. The weight loss business is a multi-billion dollar industry and diet books line bookshelves, take up space in kitchen cupboards, and collect dust on bedside tables. While each of these books works for someone, not all of these books work for everyone. And that is because we are all different. I would be remiss to assume that I know how your body works better than you do.

I have a sense of what training works, and I also know what specific tactics work for specific needs. In fact, I LOVE to figure out how to best help people! But I can only do that by fully understanding what your body does naturally, the past experiences your body has gone through, and the personal goals you want to achieve. And I can only get that information from YOU! With all of the information, we can co-create a customized plan. The goal is for you to feel good about your plan so that you enjoy sticking to it, and so the results happen as a side effect of your consistency.

Action Step: List out all of the things that make you unique. Share how you are different from everyone else and what makes you special! What would you want your coach to know about you if you were getting help with your running?

Start from Where You Are

This is about knowing your current capabilities and moving from there. It is imperative that you understand and give your body credit for its current capabilities. When you start from where you are, your progress can be incremental and allow you to reach your goal.

Think about starting to speak a foreign language. Let's take Gaelic, since it is the language of my ancestors. If someone gave me a book in Gaelic that had no pictures, no explanations, and no subtitles, I would become frustrated in a few minutes (or less) and give up. The book would go back on a shelf, and I would not pick it up again. It is not realistic to expect to be able to read it if I have no experience with that language.

All too often, I see returning runners setting up expectations that are not even close to realistic. The end result: they get frustrated, and their sneakers go back in a closet and don't get picked up again. Just like learning a language, beginning to run again can be a slow and steady process. You may have to do introductory exercises (short distances, integrate walking, etc.) in the beginning. That would be no different than a new reader using pictures and repetition to help them learn a new language.

Slow and steady wins the race. Remember, it's not about how fast you can get to your goal, it's about how long you can work toward achieving your goal. And the end line will grow and change as your capabilities do. It's about customization and personalizing YOUR growth trajectory to make your running practice something you'll love for years to come!

Action Step: Write a list of your strengths. Write an accurate description of your current running capabilities without using any words of judgment! This may be the most challenging action step, but it's the best practice!

Listen to Your Body

You know yourself best. No one knows you or your body better so make sure you listen to *you*! You've got to be a co-pilot in developing your running practice! And your practice will only become life-long if you accept the input your body shares. We are such amazing creatures! If we get scientific, we call it homeostasis, where our bodies are always trying to heal, and get back to equilibrium. When the body has difficulty, it will send out messages. When we do not hear these messages, or worse yet, ignore them, the body will rebel. It will continue to send messages, and they will get louder and louder until you HAVE to listen!

I bet you can remember a time when you had pain that you didn't listen to. In high school, I had tenderness in my shins. I would ice them and wrap them, but I continued to run. The pain turned into full-fledged shin splints and I *still* refused to listen! My body "won" when the shin splints progressed into a stress fracture of my left tibia. Had I listened, I would have only had to take a little while off. The way it turned out, I missed an entire winter track season and did not have the best spring season while I was healing. Our bodies know best. And YOU are the one who can listen and feel for the signs. No coach can feel it for you!

Action Step: Brainstorm any injuries you've ever had from sports or anything else. Have you had surgeries? Car accidents? What information do you need to remember about your body as you begin running again? This list will allow you to have compassion for your body as you begin to lace up.

Ditch Comparisons

There is absolute intention in repeating this: don't compare yourself to others! The importance of being free of judgment is worth restating over and over, because it releases your attachment to outcome and allows you to finally take action and become consistent. Let's start with the comparison to your former self. It is natural to set your upcoming goals based on where you were athletically at another time, especially for a returning runner. Thinking back to your "Glory Days" when running came easily and naturally can drive you to make a plan and say, "Hell, yeah, I can do that." Except when you give it a try and it turns out that you CAN'T do it like you used to, you drop it like a hot iron. This starts the mental game that leads to yo-yo running practices. You think because you did it before, you should just be able to get out there and do it again – and when it doesn't work out that way, instead, bam! You're sidelined.

Comparing the current you to your former self also sets you up for injury. Because you are listening to a different version of you, you may push through any pain that you're experiencing because what you're trying is something that used to be easy. But pushing through the pain will inevitably send you back to the sidelines. Forget the runner you used to be – well, don't forget her, just celebrate her and maybe use her as a role model. But don't use her as an excuse to beat yourself up or push through physical pain.

And now for comparison to others. Clients tell me *all* the time that "I'm not a real runner," or "I don't have a runner's body." Break through the stereotype of what a runner should be and get out there and RUN! Don't limit your potential by comparing yourself to what you think is a "real" runner or a "runner's body." The truth is that runners come in all shapes, sizes, and capabilities. If you don't believe me, check out Jill Angie, she has helped thousands of runners with her book, *Running with Curves*. If you find yourself believing a stereotype or coming face to face with limiting beliefs, take the time to do your three-step process so you can ditch your limiting belief and create a new affirmation.

The following are some areas you want to take into consideration when you are getting started again with your practice.

- **Your Pace:** Remember our four types of runners? They all have different paces. In fact, all runners have their "sweet spot." Finding your sweet spot may take time, but when you find it you feel like you're floating through your workout. I put pace in the customizing section because too often I see mismatched pace runners trying to work out together, and it messes up both of their routines and even lead to hating it or injury. For example, Scott and Diane both loved running when they met. It was a common bond that grew their relationship. However, after a few distance runs, it became clear that their pace was not evenly matched. He ran much faster than she did. It didn't seem like a big deal and they wanted to keep this bond so they kept running together. After a few miles, Scott would have to stop and stretch his sciatic joint because he was experiencing pain, a pain he had never had in all of his years running before. In the back of her mind, Diane knew it was because her running so much slower threw off his gait. It made her feel crappy, so she started making excuses to not go running. They needed a solution so they could both run, each at their preferred pace. They decided that they would go to the same place together, run their own workouts, and do their warm ups and cool downs together. This customization saved their running dates and kept their bodies safe.

- **Your Mileage:** Your goal will determine your mileage. Less is more when you begin and as you are working to become consistent. The last thing you want to do is push too far and not be able to get out for your next run or get sidelined by an overuse injury. You want to be in this for the long haul, so be mindful of your miles. Another part of customizing your mileage is your own personal preference. Do you prefer long distances? Short distances? The miles you cover will be representative of your preferences and goals.

- **Your Intensity:** Your intensity will also be goal-dependent. Remember the Slow & Steadies? They are noncompetitive, so they are focused on consistency rather than intensity. Some runners prefer to just get out there for the therapeutic qualities of running, and don't need or want to be doing track workouts. Other folks want to train to reach a specific time and distance goal, so track workouts will benefit their outcome. Some runners actually *love* track and interval training workouts. Again, your personal preference and goals are going to determine your workout intensity.

- **Your location:** Here where I live in Vermont, we experience all four seasons. We have to deal with snow, mud, rain, lack of sunshine, and LOTS of hills. The way I train is very different than a client in Florida, where it is hot, humid, and flat. Another consideration is elevation, especially if an event you are training for is at a different elevation from where you live. When I first got back into running, I stayed on flat and easy and then, as I began to stay more consistent and look at entering races, I would then change my location to include similar terrain. Remember, you can choose where and how to train, it's YOUR plan!

- **Your Support System:** This is a super important one to personalize! It's also a component that often gets overlooked, and is why it can seem so dang hard to stick to a plan. Are you surrounding yourself with other runners? Do the people who love you support your efforts to start running again? Will they join you? I've met a lot of runners who are "secret" runners and find it really challenging to keep going. They feel alone and unsupported. They also fear that they will be criticized for their efforts.

- I was at a networking meeting the other day, and another business owner scoffed when I mentioned I'm a running coach. He went on a spiel about how bad running is and how much he hates it. WOW! I felt like I needed a shield to repel his negativity! We can choose who we spend time with. When we're starting something new, having people who support our efforts is paramount. I came to terms with those comments by being grateful I could go back to my friends, family, clients, and running community and be loved for who I am and what I choose to do.

- In fact, here's a little melt-your-heart story. Last year I wanted to run the Smiles Turkey Trot to benefit Smiles Change Lives on Thanksgiving Day. The proceeds for this 5K run and one-mile walk go to helping children who need orthodontic work and cannot afford it. Since my birthday is near Thanksgiving, I asked my family to join me at the event in lieu of a birthday gift. I was so pleased that my mom, brother, sister-in-law, and baby niece joined my husband and me that morning. AND, a year later, my sister-in-law reached out and asked if we were all going to do the race again because she wanted to register! My heart was so warmed by this. My family is not made up of runners, but they do support me, and we all had a great time being outside and participating for a good cause. You'll be surprised where you can find support when you least expect it! And P.S., you teach people how to support you by asking!

- **Patience with Progress:** Please take the time to notice your incremental progress! No matter how small or seemingly insignificant, celebrate your consistency in getting out there. The distance will take time, the speed will take time, and you will need to practice patience with both. Runners always have ups and downs, just as anyone does. What is important is that you give yourself the time and space to grow into a practice you love. The opposite of patience is force. When you force yourself to run, consistency will be short lived. And if you force yourself to go too far too fast, you risk injury. Patience is the cornerstone for everything in this book to work. You set up the conditions for success like you would plant seeds in a garden, and you water those seeds with the utmost patience!

Finding an appropriate plan is just the first step. Then, once you listen to your body and develop your mind/body connection, you will be able to further hone in on what is good for you and what could potentially promote injury or burn-out for you. This starts the process of the Inner Game.

This is my specialty. I love to help runners find the balance between their Outer Game and Inner Game. I am fascinated by the vast similarities as well as the distinct differences among runners. I love to co-create plans with my runners and help them evolve those plans into their own custom routines. Some folks thrive on running five days a week, others on three. Some folks need cross-training, others need rest. I excel in translating your frustrations, aches and pains into specialty programming for YOU. This helps you excel at your own pace. It also helps you create a sustainable plan that you LOVE. Doesn't that sound better than where you are right now?

Running Is Community

"We awaken in others the same attitude of mind we hold toward them."
~Elbert Hubbard

You may already know this, but runners are some of the nicest, most fun-loving and colorful people on the planet! They are helpful beyond belief and want everyone in the world to experience the runner's high. Call me biased, I don't care! I have seen the best in people during my days as a young cross-country and track athlete, adult runner, New York State track official, and travel runner. I have come across thousands of people and have been inspired time after time. Running is NOT easy, and everyone out there knows what you've been through to become a runner. There is a camaraderie that I find unmatched in other sports. All you have to do is watch the Olympics. Runners are out there working their hardest to win for themselves and their country.

Do you recall what happened in the 2016 Summer Olympics in the women's 5000 meter? Two women, Abbey D'Agostino and Nikki Hamblin, collided while running and both fell. It was not a scurry to get up and beat the other runner to the line, it was a heartwarming act of kindness as D'Agostino helped Hamblin up and then Hamblin returned the favor and completely stopped to help comfort D'Agostino. That is the true character of a runner. The miles, hardships, bruises, and wins develop a deep sense of empathy. It melts the rough edges and unites. I am so happy that you are once again one of the "Nicest People on the Planet" as you get back into your running practice! Use that compassion and empathy on yourself if you need to at first, and always spread the goodness to your fellow runners and beyond.

Running has been a popular sport for many, many years. And it continues to grow as a recreational activity today. Races are popping up all over the globe to keep up with the demand for running events. Women runners who are training for half marathons make up the fastest-growing group of runners in the industry today. All you have to do is drive down the road to see people out there jogging and running. You are never alone in your practice.

Local Running Communities

If you live in an urban area, you might be able to find a local running community. There are some in rural areas also, but I have found more variety in the cities. Running stores often have group runs that you can attend, and are typically what I call "user-friendly" in that they support a variety of speeds and distance. You may also have an RRCA (Road Runners Club of America) running group in your area. These pop up in many different areas and typically offer many kinds of runs. They might do distance one day of the week and meet for track workouts on other days of the week. A third option is to check out Meetup and see if there is a local running group nearby. If you are craving a group for motivation and socializing while running, any of these options will work. Always keep in mind that your practice is custom, and while it's OK to grow into a stronger runner, forcing yourself to meet the criteria of a group will get you off track. YOU come first!

Some of my clients express that it is difficult to meet up with other runners because of scheduling or moves. I know a client who travels a lot for work, and she had a hard time meeting with her local running group because of this. She felt like she was being inconsistent, and didn't quite "fit in" because of her sporadic attendance. She never felt alienated when she did show up, but she was not able to connect in a deeper, more consistent way, which is what she craved.

Another client is a military wife and has moved multiple times to different places in the United States. Because of her travels, she has had to re-integrate many times and is tired of having to build new relationships on the fly. She wants to stay connected with her former friends in all parts of the continent.

For both of these clients, a virtual running community is a great solution. When you have access to a local, in-person, running community, that is a great option. When you have a packed schedule, travel, or move a lot and want to stay in contact with people afar, a virtual running community is a great choice.

Online Running Communities

Local running communities are great, but typically meet on a specific day at a specific time. If you're on a different schedule, it can be frustrating to make it on time or impossible to switch your schedule in order for it to be a possibility. The last thing you want is to create stress in your life trying to meet at a time that just doesn't work for you. But if you crave companionship, accountability, the social aspect of running, an online community might be perfect for you! It will give you the flexibility to run when you can fit it into your schedule, and still give you the camaraderie of a group.

If you are interested in joining a Virtual Running Club, you can go to: StartlinesGifts.com and register immediately to be a part of Running Redefined: A Virtual Running Club designed for runners just like you!

If running with others truly isn't your thing, there are many other ways to feel connected to community. Charity running is a great example, and helps others while feeding your soul. There are many benefit runs out there that use your entry fee for a great cause. Sometimes you can directly help individuals, organizations, or large causes. By participating in these events, you are helping your community. You might also opt to support someone else who is in training and raising money for an event. This will help the cause and reinforce someone else's running practice.

Lastly, I want to share how my in-laws make running and walking a contribution to their community. Once a week, my father-in-law, who is still running four days a week at the age of 76, brings a bag and picks up garbage along the roadside. It is a country road and sees its fair share of litter over the course of the week. My mother-in-law also picks up trash once a week while walking, and we neighbors are grateful. I know that I will continue the tradition when they tire of it and do my part for our local community.

The bottom line is, running is so much more than just you. Even if you are just doing it for yourself, you make an impact on other people. You become a role model for others and inspire them to take their health into their own hands.

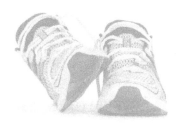

Chapter 8

Overcoming Obstacles

"It's your life. Rise up and run with it."
~Sarah Richardson

I've just tossed a lot of information at you. I hope you can see where traditional training plans fall short, and how you may have stalled out because no one taught you about the Inner Game of running and how to effectively deal with it. I hope you can fully appreciate the Outer Game AND Inner Game of running, because when you're missing one or the other, consistency will become a challenge. I have the upmost confidence that you will be able to use the information in this book to get your groove again. I hope that you are no longer confused about why you have been feeling so frustrated and disheartened when trying to lace up. I hope that you are DONE beating yourself up and comparing yourself to who you used to be.

Remember, you're reading this because your goal is to start running again and fall in love with your practice. If you've made it this far in this book, I KNOW you are serious and you've tried EVERYTHING already! You want to be empowered by your choices and to create a practice that lasts a lifetime. We are talking longevity here.

Knowing what you now know, are you ready to start running consistently? Are you ready to work on your relationship with running? Is it time for you to fall in love with your practice again? If so, think of it as if you are entering a new relationship. You have just redefined what running could look like for you. You are looking for that love affair with running, and the physical, mental, and emotional healing benefits running provides. And you want it to be sustainable. You don't ever want to feel "lazy" or "unmotivated" again, because those stories are not true in the first place!

You have learned about the Outer and Inner Games of running and how they make up the foundation of a running program. They set the groundwork so that you can be fully prepared and fully appreciate the effort you're putting into the relationship. You'll need to be patient, put in the effort, and show up consistently, knowing that it's totally worth it. You now have the tools to nurture your Inner Athlete.

You learned about the four pillars that support a thriving, sustainable, consistent and enjoyable practice. Ensuring that your practice is therapeutic, experiential, custom, and communal will deepen your relationship with running and make it more and more irresistible every day. You'll wind up feeling antsy when you miss a day, and excited for your next run rather than feeling frustrated that you put it off another day.

With this information, I hope that you dig in, work on the exercises, and take action. Leave your frustration behind and reconnect with your body on a personal, physical, and spiritual level. Your Inner Athlete directed you to pick up this book. She's telling you she's ready. Only you have the ability to commit.

Remember, I had to choose health, and I chose running as my way to achieve it. You, too, can do the same.

While this book gives you all of the tools you'll need to set up your own success, you might be someone who wants support along the way and needs personal accountability. If you try to implement this plan and you still find yourself frustrated and avoiding your practice, it might be time to reach out for help. If going at it alone leaves you with questions and has kept you in a cycle of self-doubt, it's time to reach out. For those looking to follow a proven training program, I've got just what you need. Unlike training programs that prepare you just for a specific distance, I help clients put their own plan into place, one that goes beyond a single finish line. My hope, and I believe your hope, too, is to run forever. You're in it for the long haul and want this to be so much more than another yo-yo training plan. I assure you it is. Clients nation wide have achieved success using this program.

When I work with clients like you, I spend time setting your foundation specific to your needs with the Outer and Inner Games. You will feel confident knowing that you are well prepared to start training again from focusing on your Outer Game. As you navigate your Inner Game, your consistency will grow, your frustration will fade, and your self-trust will build. You will feel excited as you recognize your new habits. You will learn to say YES to you, embrace and empower your body, and ditch self-sabotage.

Together you and I will build up your pillars, and when they are in place, you will experience the consistency you have been craving all along. You will condition your body and optimize your potential during our weeks together. If you're ready to exponentially boost your efforts and get to your goal of being consistent more quickly, let's talk: email me at Sarah@ RiseAndShine.Run and be sure to pick up your resources at StartlinesGifts.com.

It is my deepest hope that you love your running practice again and lace up for a lifetime! I truly wish for you to be happy and healthy through your practice of running. It has done wonders for my life, and I hope it does wonders for yours! Running is always so much more than just a form of exercise. It has a way of shaping our lives into something bigger. When you run, you are able to run your life in ways that might not have been possible. Take pride in yourself for taking this first step and reading this book. Bring forth your passion, take charge of your health, and find yourself on the start line of your future.

As a fellow runner, I warmly welcome you back to the sport and hope you find Peace, Sanity and Love in your practice. May you lace up for a lifetime!

Shine on,
Coach Sarah

Acknowledgements

There are so many people I want to thank. This book has been a growth experience on so many levels. I want to first and foremost thank my husband, Mike Richardson, for believing in me and for supporting me every step of the way. Without your excited and sometimes blatant questioning, I might have given up. And of course, thank you for being such an inspiration and role model for consistency and dedication. I love you so much!

To my mind, body, and soul: I am grateful beyond words. Without being injured – and recovering – this idea would have never sparked. I am thankful for my dark times, which led me to the light. Thank you, body and mind, for your deep connection and for going the distance with me. You are truly amazing!

To all of my former and current coaches, Mr. Farber, Mr. Williams, Mr. Schoppman, and Danny Dreyer, I would not be the runner I am today without your kind guidance, continued encouragement and belief in me. To the Chi Running community, I am honored and blessed to be a part of this supportive group. I am an eternal student!

To Julie Sullivan, your kind words while "on the bus" taught me to connect with writing in a whole new way. You gave me permission to write from the heart. You taught me to not take myself so seriously, and that no written work is ever truly perfect.

To Angela, you have rocked my world during this process. Your ability to facilitate this process is legendary. Your gift to me was pointed guidance, tough love, and accountability. But most of all, you taught me to be me. Thank you for creating the space to let this shy author spill it out. This process has empowered me in many ways and truly helped me find my voice. And Maggie McReynolds, your feedback, comments, and clarity explaining the editing process were priceless. There is no way I could have sharpened my manuscript to this point without your expert guidance. Thank you from the bottom of my heart.

To the Morgan James Publishing team: Special thanks to David Hancock, CEO & Founder for believing in me and my message. To my Author Relations Manager, Gayle West, thanks for making the process seamless and easy. Many more thanks to everyone else, but especially Jim Howard, Bethany Marshall, and Nickcole Watkins.

To Leanne Phillips and Maureen Posten, all I can say is OMG! Thank you a million times over. You have believed in the concept of my book from day one, and put the program to the test! Your genuine interest and belief that I'm on the right path is met with gratitude and love.

To my fellow runners, past, current and future clients, you have given me my purpose. I have so much gratitude for each and every one of you, and am inspired by your stories and experiences. I am humbled and honored to be of service to you.

And to ALL of my friends and family, I would not be the person I am today if it weren't for you. I count my blessings to be surrounded and supported by you all. Thank you so very much!

About the Author

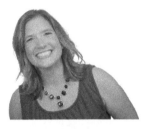

Sarah Richardson, M.S., M.Ed. is a certified distance running coach through RRCA and Chi Walking/Chi Running® Instructor through Chi Living. She is an outdoor enthusiast, world traveler, and Racecation facilitator. Her business, Rise And Shine, designs custom training programs that provide the external components involved with running and fully address the emotional and internal components that have trapped frustrated runners in yo-yo training cycles. Sarah knows that running brings joy to life, and knows the hard work it takes to get back into the sport. After a four-year hiatus from running due to an injury, she found herself frustrated and fed up at her inconsistency and lack of commitment to the sport. Now back to running multiple distance races per year in different places around the world, Sarah has made it her life's work to help struggling runners find the daily discipline to take back their power and honor their runner within. Sarah lives and trains in Vermont, and is happily married to her husband Mike.

Thank You

Thank you for taking the time to read this book. Although you are finished reading, this is not the end! In fact it's just the beginning. The exercises and examples in my book are your first step toward getting off of those Sidelines and back onto those Start lines.

To continue your momentum, visit StartlinesGifts.com to gather up your free gifts. You will learn more about ditching your frustration and lacing up for a lifetime with love. You will have immediate access to the Sustainable Running Toolkit and Running Redefined: A Virtual Running Club

For additional contact information:

Sarah@RiseAndShine.Run
(802) 522-3000
www.facebook.com/RiseAndShine.Run
twitter.com/RiseAndShineRun
www.instagram.com/riseandshinerun/

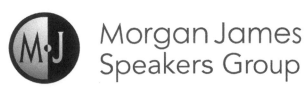

Morgan James
Speakers Group

We connect Morgan James published authors with live and online events and audiences who will benefit from their expertise.

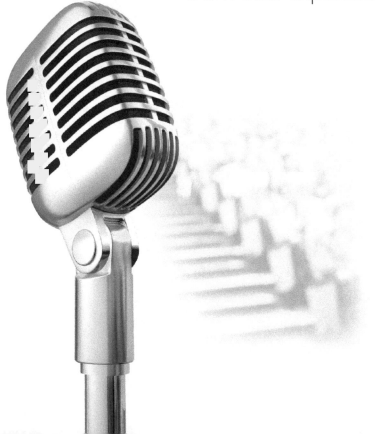

Morgan James makes all of our titles available
through the Library for All Charity Organization.

www.LibraryForAll.org

CPSIA information can be obtained
at www.ICGtesting.com
Printed in the USA
BVHW01s2238100118
505035BV00001B/1/P